Cognitive-Behavioral Treatment for Adult Survivors of Childhood Trauma

Cognitive-Behavioral Treatment for Adult Survivors of Childhood Trauma

Imagery Rescripting and Reprocessing

Mervin R. Smucker, Ph.D.
Constance V. Dancu, Ph.D.

A JASON ARONSON BOOK

ROWMAN & LITTLEFIELD PUBLISHERS, INC.
Lanham • Boulder • New York • Toronto • Oxford

A JASON ARONSON BOOK

ROWMAN & LITTLEFIELD PUBLISHERS, INC.

Published in the United States of America
by Rowman & Littlefield Publishers, Inc.
A wholly owned subsidiary of The Rowman & Littlefield Publishing Group, Inc.
4501 Forbes Boulevard, Suite 200, Lanham, Maryland 20706
www.rowmanlittlefield.com

PO Box 317
Oxford
OX2 9RU, UK

Copyright © 1999 by Jason Aronson Inc.
First Rowman & Littlefield Edition 2005

All rights reserved. No part of this publication may be reproduced, stored in a retrieval system, or transmitted in any form or by any means, electronic, mechanical, photocopying, recording, or otherwise, without the prior permission of the publisher.

British Library Cataloguing in Publication Information Available

Library of Congress Cataloging-in-Publication Data

Smucker, Mervin R.
   Cognitive-behavioral treatment for adult survivors of childhood trauma : imagery rescripting and reprocessing / Mervin R. Smucker, Constance V. Dancu.
      p. cm.— (New directions in cognitive-behavior therapy)
   Includes bibliographical references and index.
   ISBN 0-7657-0213-4
   1. Adult child abuse victims—Rehabilitation. 2. Cognitive therapy. 3. Desensitization (Psychotherapy) I. Dancu, Constance V. III. Title. IV. Series.
   RC569.5.C55S65 1999
   616.85'822390651—dc21   98-53686

Printed in the United States of America

∞™ The paper used in this publication meets the minimum requirements of American National Standard for Information Sciences—Permanence of Paper for Printed Library Materials, ANSI/NISO Z39.48-1992.

This book is dedicated
To Jonathan Stoltzfus Smucker
and
Ann, Elizabeth, Jonathan, Julia, and David,
with love and appreciation for your
patience and understanding
M.R.S.

To George, Connie, John, and Chris,
with love and deep appreciation
for your support
C.V.D.

Contents

Foreword   xi
by Robert L. Leahy

Preface   xv

Acknowledgments   xix

Part I
Childhood Trauma and Its Aftermath

1. Introduction   3

    • Childhood Sexual Abuse • Trauma-Related Beliefs and Schemata • Traumagenic Schemas and the Link to PTSD • PTSD: Characteristics and Symptoms • The Nature of Traumatic Memory • Type I vs. Type II Trauma • Information-Processing Models of PTSD • Indicators of Emotional Processing • Transforming Trauma into Words: A Critical Component of Healing

2. A Conceptual Overview   19

    • Clinical Applications of Imagery: An Historical Overview • Imagery Applications Within a

Cognitive-Behavioral Context • Attachment Theory and Its Relevance • Object Relations Theory and the Role of Introjects • Primary vs. Secondary Cognitive Processing • Goals of IRRT

Part II
Imagery Rescripting and Reprocessing Therapy

3. Pretreatment Evaluation 33
    • Recommended Inclusion Criteria • Recommended Exclusion Criteria • Concomitant Use of Medication • Introducing IRRT to the Patient

4. Exposure, Rescripting, and Self-Nurturing Imagery 39
    • Session 1: Beginning Treatment • Presenting the Treatment Rationale • Introducing Subjective Units of Distress (SUDs) • Imaginal Exposure: Reexperiencing the Traumatic Event • Mastery Imagery: Rescripting the Traumatic Imagery • Developing Adult-Nurturing-Child Imagery • Administering the Post-Imagery Questionnaire • Processing and Debriefing • Assessing Self-Calming and Self-Soothing Abilities • Contracting for Safety • Homework • Sessions 2 Through 8 • Guidelines for Crisis

5. Self-Nurturing Imagery Only 81
    • Sessions 9 Through 13

6. A Higher Order Cognitive/Linguistic Processing 95
    • Sessions 14 Through 18 • Posttreatment Assessment • Relapse Prevention/Maintenance Sessions

Part III
Special Considerations

7. Imagery Rescripting Format for Each Additional Recurring Traumatic Memory — 125

8. When Difficulties Arise During the Imagery Session — 133

9. When IRRT Is Not Indicated: Alternate Cognitive-Behavioral Treatment Options — 141
   - Treating Partial PTSD-Related Symptoms

Part IV
Case Studies

10. Case Example 1: One-Session IRRT — 153

11. Case Example 2: Eight-Session IRRT — 159

12. Case Example 3: Extended IRRT with Higher Order Cognitive/Linguistic Processing — 181

Appendices — 219
   - Appendix A: Treatment Rationale • Appendix B: The Post-Imagery Questionnaire • Appendix C: Therapist Record • Appendix D: Homework Record • Appendix E: Traumatic Flashback Incident Record

References — 241

Index — 251

Foreword

In recent years, there has been an increasing interest in the diagnosis and treatment of those who have suffered earlier sexual, physical, or psychological abuse. This book is a significant advance in the treatment of individuals with Post-Traumatic Stress Syndrome resulting from early childhood abuse.

The authors have provided an integrative theoretical model of abuse by drawing on cognitive, behavioral, psychodynamic, and attachment theories. Many who have suffered from abuse use avoidance and escape as strategies for immediately reducing discomfort. Unfortunately, some therapists, family, and friends of abused individuals exhort the victim to "put the abuse out of your mind" or to "stop thinking about it." As the authors indicate, these attempts at cognitive avoidance only perpetuate the underlying belief that one cannot handle the memory of the abuse, thereby maintaining the need to avoid or escape from the memory.

Since many more individuals actually suffer abuse than develop PTSD, the theoretical overview in the first section of the book is a helpful place for us to begin. The cognitive and emotional processing of abuse is essential in the emergence of later clinical phenomena. In my treatment of a woman who had suffered two separate experiences of abuse, it was interesting to note which abusive experience was linked with her current problem (dissociative disorder). One experience occurred when she was threatened at knifepoint and compelled to have sex. Recognizing that she needed to maintain clarity in thinking to protect herself from being killed, she remained alert and calm. This did not lead to traumatic sequelae. However, her experience of being sexually molested by her father led to her reliance on dissociation, which resulted in the persistence through adulthood of dissociation whenever she had intercourse. In her case, the emotional processing of the abuse, as well as the cognitive meaning, differed. For her, the incestuous abuse was not reprocessed and her "meaning" for the abuse was that she was disgusting.

Smucker and Dancu provide a detailed, yet concise treatment manual approach in the second part of this book. Here they indicate that reactivating the initial memories of abuse allows the therapist and the patient to elicit and examine the negative cognitions associated with the abuse. One goal of treatment is to assist the patient in developing *mastery imagery*—that is, mastery of the sense of being a victim. They urge the patient to develop an image in which the outcome of the abuse is "rescripted" so that the patient feels more like a thriver than a victim. This approach empowers the patient, who may have heretofore felt like she was helpless and disgusting. Furthermore, the patient is helped to write processing letters to the perpetrator of the abuse or to those who remained in silent collaboration. These acts of assertion further empower the patient to be a thriver. The authors demonstrate how to challenge the patient's negative thoughts, assumptions, and schemas that arise from the abuse experiences. For example, the patient who believes she is worthless because she was sexually molested during childhood is asked if she would use this same standard to judge others who have been abused. Finally, the patient is assisted in finding what can be learned or even what can come of her experience that is positive. Smucker and

Dancu draw on Viktor Frankl's provocative experiences as a prisoner in a concentration camp to evoke the meaning that one can draw from these events.

Case studies bring to life the use of these techniques and conceptualizations, illustrating how imagery rescripting can be utilized, even within a single session. One is struck by the directness and compassion the therapists use when employing the techniques. My experience using imagery rescripting techniques has taught me the necessity of adapting a collaborative and supportive role in dealing with the victimized patient. Yet, one does not want to reinforce an infantilized view of the victim in which she always remains an injured child. Imagery rescripting and reprocessing therapy allows the therapist to join with the patient by identifying the negative personal meanings attached to the abuse and empowering the victim to overcome the memories that reside for years in her personal schemas.

This book will prove valuable to clinicians who want to employ active, compassionate, sensible, and empowering therapy for victims of childhood sexual abuse. The clarity of the presentation, the detailed and concise treatment manual approach, and the hands-on case studies will give the reader powerful tools for conceptualizing and modifying the effects of early abuse.

Robert L. Leahy
June 1999

Preface

This book is based on the integration of our theoretical perspectives and our many years of research and clinical experience in working with adult victims of sexual assault and survivors of childhood sexual and physical abuse. The number of women who are sexually victimized as children or adults is shocking, and many seek professional help from a gynecologist, primary health physician, or mental health clinician. How the professional responds can make the difference between the patient's starting on a path to recovery or continuing to suffer. The case history may be complex and may include problems with substance abuse, self-mutilating behavior, suicide ideation or attempts, eating disorders, dissociative reactions, depression, sexual dysfunctions, and serious interpersonal problems.

The treatment program described here addresses the chronic posttraumatic stress disorder (PTSD) symptoms and related problems experienced by many adult survivors of childhood trauma. We have integrated the prolonged imaginal exposure treatment program, which has been systematically studied for a number of years with victims of rape and nonsexual crime, with imaginal rescripting, which replaces the recurring traumatic images with mastery imagery. This book provides a comprehensive description of the integrated cognitive-behavioral treatment program that can be implemented with survivors (male and female) of childhood sexual, physical, and emotional trauma.

The authors' paths initially crossed in the 1990s, when Edna B. Foa, Ph.D., was invited by Mervin R. Smucker, Ph.D., to present the results of the National Institute of Mental Health (NIMH)-funded treatment study at the Medical College of Wisconsin of female adult victims of rape.

Following an exchange of ideas on Dr. Foa's work, as well as on the clinical work that Dr. Smucker was initiating with adult survivors of CSA using imagery rescripting interventions, Drs. Foa and Smucker began to discuss the possibility of doing collaborative work with this population. At the same time, Constance Dancu, Ph.D., had initiated a treatment program for survivors of childhood sexual abuse using a combined treatment of prolonged imaginal exposure and stress inoculation training (PE/SIT). The three authors subsequently met at the Medical College of Pennsylvania in Philadelphia to further develop a cognitive-behavioral treatment program, which involved establishing a pilot study designed to evaluate the efficacy of PE/SIT and imagery rescripting with adult CSA survivors suffering from posttraumatic stress disorder.

SUMMARY OF THE CLINICAL OUTCOME PILOT STUDY

The results of the pilot study were very favorable to both imagery rescripting and PE/SIT (Dancu et al., in preparation). Briefly, the study consisted of twelve subjects (six subjects in each treatment group), all of whom met *DSM* criteria for PTSD at pretreatment. At the completion of treatment, all subjects in both treatment groups showed a significant reduction in PTSD-related symptoms, and no longer did any subject in either treatment group meet criteria for PTSD. These positive results for both groups were maintained at three months and six months follow-up.

Several empirical studies currently being conducted at the Medical College of Wisconsin with victims of industrial accidents suffering from PTSD offer considerable evidence that imagery rescripting is more effective than prolonged imaginal exposure in treating PTSD when there is a perceived perpetrator—that is, when the victim perceives an individual or an object (e.g., a machine) as the culprit for the accident (Grunert, Rusch, et al., in preparation). Interestingly, where no perpetrator is assumed or perceived, prolonged imaginal exposure combined with in vivo exposure appears to be the most effective treatment with this clinical population (Grunert, Weis, and Rusch, in preparation).

The results of these studies are indeed encouraging, though they are by no means definitive, and further outcome research is needed to corroborate these findings. While it is crucial that clinicians be cautious about using or promoting new treatments that have not been adequately tested, it would seem irresponsible to tell adult survivors of childhood trauma suffering from PTSD that they cannot be treated at this time because definitive outcome treatment studies have not yet been completed with this clinical population.

Acknowledgments

To all the courageous childhood sexual abuse survivors who, through sharing with us their pain and suffering, have helped us to develop this treatment program.

M. R. S. and C. V. D.

During the past seven years, I have been greatly enriched by clinicians and students attending my imagery rescripting classes and training workshops. I have been especially inspired by my encounters with European friends and colleagues. A special thanks to Janet Feigenbaum, Rod Holland, Vartouhi Ohanian, and Louise Sharp in London, whose continued feedback and unwavering encouragement during my initial lecture tours in England helped to keep me energized and on track. A heartfelt thanks to my colleagues and good friends Deborah Meirs and Maxine Cresswell in Northern Ireland, whose generous support and stimulating feedback over the years have been an enormous inspiration to me and my work. Thanks also to my German colleagues, Dirk and Toni Zimmer, for the valuable support and critical feedback they have offered me over the past decade, including the many hours of help with translating my imagery rescripting lectures into German. A very special thanks to my Swiss colleagues and cherished friends Uli Junghan, Monika Buergi, and Gregor Berger, whose willingness over the past several years to spend enormous blocks of their time in debate and discussion provided me with unparalleled inspiration and encouragement to pursue my clinical intuitions. A heartfelt thanks to Henck van Bilsen and Lynn Norris in New Zealand for their undaunting support, encouragement, and insightful feedback from their early clinical experimentations with imagery rescripting that contributed significantly to the further development and refinement of the procedure.

I have also received much encouragement from Donald Meichenbaum, a resourceful colleague and leading PTSD expert, whose generous support and stimulating feedback over the past decade have been invaluable to me. Special appreciation is extended to Robert Leahy for encouraging me to write this book and the support he offered throughout the process.

I am especially grateful to Edna Foa for her crucial support in the early stages of this project, for sponsoring the imagery rescripting clinical outcome pilot study at the Medical College of Pennsylvania and for being a co-author on several of the earlier imagery rescripting publications. A special thanks also to Jan Niederee for her contributions early on as a co-author of several articles on imagery rescripting, and to Amy Ridley Meyers for her enthusiastic support and assistance in helping to refine the clinical application of imagery rescripting over the years.

A very special thanks to Aaron T. Beck, my original cognitive therapy mentor, for all the hours of rich intellectual stimulation, debate, and training he offered during the six formative years I spent at the University of Pennsylvania Center for Cognitive Therapy in Philadelphia. It was he who first showed me how to conceptualize a case from a cognitive perspective. He also taught me the Socratic method, which I have found to be a most useful tool in enhancing the quality of human dialogue.

I would like to express my deepest thanks and appreciation to the members of the Medical College of Wisconsin Imagery Rescripting Research Group (my professional family): Brad Grunert, Ann Huebner, Robert Mendelsohn, Mark Rusch, Pam Shapson, Susan Stacy, and Jo Weis, who have collaborated with me, inspired me, and provided extremely useful feedback on my endeavors to make sense of the clinical phenomena I was observing. A very special thanks also to Pam Shapson for the many hours she contributed in the clinical application of imagery rescripting, her intuitive and creative insights, and the personal support she offered during the latter stages of this work.

A very warm, heartfelt thanks to Mary Krentz for her enthusiastic support, insightful feedback, and assistance in the early conceptual phases of imagery rescripting. I am eternally grateful to Mary for the countless hours of tireless energy she put forth in reviewing, organizing, critiquing, and transcribing the numerous imagery rescripting videotapes that were essential to the completion of this project.

I wish to thank my patients for having the courage to share with me recurring painful images of their traumatic pasts as they struggled to find healing from and meaning in their pain and suffering. A very special thank you to Connie Taylor for all that she has taught me over the past five years about healing, recovery, and the courageous search for meaning in a highly traumatic past.

Finally, I would like to thank the members of my family, without whose support this project would have been unthinkable. A very warm, heartfelt thanks to my parents, Mary and Robert, for always being there when I needed them and whose unconditional love, support, and acceptance over the years fostered a home environment conducive to intellectual exploration and growth. I am also grateful to my parents-in-law,

John and Beulah, for their steadfast support over the past twenty years and for being academic role models par excellence. I would like to thank my children, Elizabeth, Jonathan, Julia, and David, for their patience, inspiration, and love throughout this project.

Lastly, I would like to express my deepest gratitude and appreciation to my wife and best friend, Ann, for the rich intellectual stimulation and emotional support that she has provided throughout all aspects of his project. In addition to being a full-time academic and an exceptional mother to our children, she is my most respected and cherished colleague.

Mervin R. Smucker, Ph.D.

A very special thank you to my husband, George Dancu, for his confidence in me, dedication, and loving support throughout my career. I would also like to thank a number of excellent professors, supervisors, and colleagues who have provided me opportunities, training, and support in my career as a clinician/researcher.

My roots in behavior therapy were developed and formulated by Joseph Wolpe, M.D., Edna B. Foa, Ph.D., Ralph M. Turner, Ph.D., and Debora Phillips, D.O. During my internship at the Behavior Therapy Unit, Department of Psychiatry at Temple University School of Medicine, the late Dr. Wolpe was an inspiration. He fostered dedication to research, behavioral analysis, case formulation, and to providing a high quality of creative mental health services to each patient. He is greatly missed, but his influence will live on in his work and in the many professionals who follow in his footsteps. My heartfelt thanks to Dr. Wolpe for his outstanding contributions.

Dr. Ralph Turner provided me with an excellent role model for a supervisor. I appreciated his consistent and dedicated clinical supervision during my internship and his ongoing support throughout my career. I frequently reflect upon Dr.

Debora Phillips's creative conceptualization and treatment interventions when I work with difficult cases.

Thank you to Thomas Detre, M.D., who launched my career at the University of Pittsburgh School of Medicine and the Western Psychiatric Institute and Clinic, and provided me with the opportunities to develop my research, clinical, and administrative skills during my eight-year tenure.

Special appreciation is extended to Edna Foa, Ph.D., who influenced my early development as a behavior therapist during my internship, and later was instrumental in providing me with the opportunity to pursue my research/clinical interests in the area of trauma. My initial experience with Dr. Foa as a teacher-supervisor and later as a colleague have spanned a number of years and provided me with opportunities to continue to develop as a professional.

Finally, I would like to thank my colleagues at the Center for Cognitive and Behavior Therapy for their support and for being instrumental in allowing my dreams to come true with respect to the establishment of a mental health center that provides training, supervision, and outstanding therapeutic interventions for our patients.

Constance V. Dancu, Ph.D.

PART I

CHILDHOOD TRAUMA AND ITS AFTERMATH

1
Introduction

CHILDHOOD SEXUAL ABUSE

In recent years, a growing body of literature has attested to the prevalence of childhood sexual abuse and its long-term deleterious effects on victims. The National Women's Study (National Victim Center 1992) reported that one out of eight women in the United States has been the victim of forcible rape during her lifetime and that over 60 percent of these assaults occurred during childhood and adolescence (29 percent before age 11, 32 percent between ages 11 and 17). Recent figures indicate that between 156,000 and 300,000 children are identified each year as victims of sexual abuse (Beutler et al. 1994), although there are no doubt many more that go unreported.

Despite some conflicting views on the psychological impact of childhood sexual abuse (CSA), there is substantial evidence that CSA victims suffer from serious short-term and long-term effects (Briere 1992, 1997b, Bryer et al. 1987, Finkelhor et al. 1989, O'Neill and Gupta 1991). As noted by Briere (1992), childhood abuse significantly disrupts a child's development, resulting in the development of primitive coping strategies and the creation of cognitive distortions of self, relationships, and one's future. Symptoms frequently observed among sexually abused children include an increased incidence of depression (Lipovsky et al. 1989), heightened anxiety (Gomes-Schwartz et al. 1990), sleep disturbance, nightmares, school difficulties, social withdrawal, sexualized behaviors, frequent outbursts of anger or other acting-out behaviors (Friedrich 1991, Kolko et al. 1988), and a variety of somatic symptoms including stomachaches, headaches, and vulnerability to disease (Kimerling and Calhoun 1994).

Clinical phenomena frequently observed with adult survivors of CSA include depression, anxiety and panic disorders, chronic sleep disturbance, nightmares, flashbacks, dissociation, interpersonal and sexual difficulties, substance abuse, eating disorders, self-abusive behaviors, and suicidality (Briere 1992, Browne and Finkelhor 1986, Coons et al. 1989, Courtois 1988, Goodwin and Talwar 1989, Russell 1986, Walker 1994). Long-term psychological effects of childhood sexual abuse often include chronic feelings of worthlessness, guilt, self-blame, self-hatred, vulnerability, generalized mistrust of others, and a pervasive sense of powerlessness, hopelessness, and despair (Bagley and Ramsay 1986, Briere and Runtz 1992, Herman 1992, Janoff-Bulman 1985, Jehu 1991, McCann et al. 1988, Smucker et al. 1995).

TRAUMA-RELATED BELIEFS AND SCHEMATA

A number of authors have attributed these long-term deleterious effects of childhood sexual abuse to fundamental beliefs about self, world, and relationships that became part of the child's cognitive schemata when the traumas occurred and have continued to be reinforced by subsequent experience. According to Piaget's theory of human adaptation and cognitive development (Rosen 1989), children (as well as adults) attempt to make sense of their life experiences and adapt to their environment via two cognitive processes: assimilation and accommodation.

The process of assimilation with childhood abuse victims may involve altering or distorting the abuse in order to cognitively fit it into already-existing schematic structures. Children with abusive caregivers often develop negative self-views or self-schemas, making internal attributions and blaming themselves for their beatings: "I get beaten because I'm such a bad kid." Thus, if a child already has developed negative self-schemas, attempts to assimilate the experience of incest could be manifested by such cognitions as: "Daddy wouldn't do something like that." "It must have been my fault." "It must have happened because I'm such a bad person." "Maybe it wasn't really so bad after all." "Maybe it didn't really happen."

By contrast, the process of accommodation involves altering existing schemas and forming new schematic structures or categories, in order to take in the new information and incorporate it into a new cognitive frame. Thus, if a child has had relatively positive self-schemas prior to the abuse, attempts to accommodate the experience of incest may involve disrupting or altering previous schemata relating to perceptions of self and others such that a schema of powerlessness may become dominant; a sense of relative safety may be replaced by chronic feelings of vulnerability; feelings of relative trust toward others may be replaced by a generalized and pervasive mistrust of others; a sense of connectedness with one's caregivers may be replaced by feelings of aloneness and emotional abandonment; feelings of worthiness may be replaced by feelings of inherent unworthiness and unlovability. Finally, a positive sense of self may be replaced with a view of self as being bad, stigmatized, and evil. Moreover, such negative views of self and others may then become repeatedly reinforced by continued abuse experiences throughout childhood and adolescence, such that by early adulthood these beliefs become generalized and form the core of the individual's schematic beliefs, which are not only quite maladaptive, but extremely difficult to modify as well.

The schematic disruptions that children experience following the trauma of sexual abuse have been increasingly recognized and corroborated by a number of writers in recent years. Finkelhor and Browne (1985) emphasized the tremendous impact that sexual abuse has on a child's self-concept and worldview, and referred to the resultant schematic disruptions as "traumagenic dynamics" that contribute to postabuse pathology. Janoff-Bulman (1989) attributed most posttrauma pathology of childhood sexual abuse survivors to a shattering of the victim's self-worth, personal invulnerability, and fundamental assumptions concerning the benevolence and meaningfulness of the world. McCann and Pearlman (1990) noted that disruptions in schemas often become pathological in core areas of safety, trust, power, esteem, intimacy, independence, and frame of reference. Jehu (1988) noted a number of self-denigratory core beliefs that frequently result from the experience of childhood sexual abuse, including beliefs of worthlessness, badness, inadequacy, inferiority, stigmatization, and subordination of rights. Smucker and Niederee (1995) identified pathogenic, abuse-related schemas of powerlessness, mistrust, abandonment, worthlessness, self-blame, inherent badness, and unlovability as being particularly prevalent in traumatized childhood sexual abuse survivors.

TRAUMAGENIC SCHEMAS AND THE LINK TO PTSD

According to schema theory (e.g., Beck et al. 1990, Guidano 1987, Guidano and Liotti 1983, Young 1994), once the abuse-related, trauma-based schemas are in place and solidified, they act as powerful cognitive templates that filter and organize mental processes and significantly influence how the victim perceives, interprets, encodes, and recalls subsequent events. The continued activation of affectively charged, abuse-related schemas (e.g., schemas of powerlessness, vulnerability, worthlessness, unlovability, inherent badness, and abandonment) may then serve not only to emotionally overwhelm CSA victims and keep them in a perpetual state of perceived victimization long after the abuse itself has ceased, but also to lay the foundation for the onset of a chronic PTSD. Traumagenic schemas may be triggered by internal cognitive stimuli (e.g., dreams, flashbacks, emotions, visual or verbal associations) or external, environmental stimuli (e.g., odors, a scary movie, a frightening encounter or event).

The PTSD link to these abuse-related schemas is corroborated by recent research findings suggesting that the psychological sequelae experienced by many survivors of childhood sexual abuse are consistent with chronic or delayed onset of PTSD (Blake-White and Kline 1985, Briere and Runtz 1987, Coons et al. 1989, Donaldson and Gardner 1985, Jehu 1991, O'Neill and Gupta 1991, van der Kolk 1987; also see North et al. [1994] for a discussion of comorbidity and PTSD). Increasingly, clinicians and researchers are reporting the delayed onset of clinical PTSD symptoms emerging with adult survivors of CSA. One study by O'Neill and Gupta (1991) reported a mean of 10.7 years from the cessation of abuse to the onset of PTSD symptoms in a clinical population of twenty-six female CSA survivors.

For many adult CSA survivors, the trauma-based powerlessness schema appears to form the nucleus of their PTSD syndrome, leaving them in a state of functional "paralysis." A frequently observed behavioral manifestation of a PTSD sufferer's powerlessness schema is the victim's perceived helplessness vis-à-vis his or her recurring abuse memory flashbacks. The notion that victims may have internal resources available, albeit not yet accessed, to gain mastery and control over their recurring abuse flashbacks would be incompatible with their powerlessness schema. Thus, it is the maladaptive behavioral manifestations of the abuse victim's long-standing powerlessness schema that, directly or indirectly, become the initial primary target of cognitive-behavioral PTSD-focused treatments (Smucker 1997).

PTSD: CHARACTERISTICS AND SYMPTOMS

According to the fourth edition of the *Diagnostic and Statistical Manual of Mental Disorders* (*DSM-IV*; American Psychiatric Association 1994), an individual exposed to a traumatic event may develop PTSD if

1. the person experienced, witnessed, or was confronted with an event or events that involve actual or threatened death or serious injury, or a threat to the physical integrity of self or others, and

2. the person's response involved intense fear, helplessness, or horror. [pp. 427–428]

The following symptoms, if present for at least one month, are characteristic of a PTSD syndrome: (1) recurrent, intrusive distressing recollections of a traumatic event (e.g., recurring images, flashbacks, nightmares) accompanied by intense affective distress; (2) avoidance of stimuli associated with the trauma and/or numbing of general responsiveness; and (3) increased arousal (e.g., hypervigilance, exaggerated startle response, sleep disturbance, irritability). All of these symptoms have been reported in the literature as long-term deleterious effects of childhood sexual abuse, which suggests that PTSD is very much a part of the clinical profile presented by adults who have been sexually abused in childhood.

The following PTSD subtypes are also delineated in the *DSM-IV*: acute PTSD, when the duration of symptoms is less than three months; chronic PTSD, when the duration of symptoms is three months or more; and delayed-onset of PTSD, when the onset of the PTSD symptoms occurs at least six months after the traumatic event. According to *DSM-IV*, PTSD tends to be more severe and longer lasting when the traumatic event is of human design (e.g., sexual abuse, physical torture, or war atrocities, in contrast to accidents or natural disasters, such as floods or earthquakes).

THE NATURE OF TRAUMATIC MEMORY

Numerous writers have observed that traumatic memories appear to be encoded and accessed differently from nontraumatic memories. In their work with traumatized children and adults, van der Kolk and van der Hart (1991) observed that recurring traumatic memories involve primary sensory stimuli (e.g., visual, auditory, kinesthetic, and tactile). They describe the raw, unprocessed nature of traumatic memories as follows:

> Trauma stops the chronological clock and fixes the traumatic moment in memory and imagination. Such traumatic memories are not usually altered by the mere passage of time. These traumatic memories become fixed and the intense vehement emotions interfere with their natural processing. These traumatic memories are not organized on a linguistic line. [p. 447]

Van der Kolk and van der Hart (1989, 1991) concluded that, in contrast to nontraumatic memories, traumatic memories (1) lack verbal narrative and context, (2) are state dependent, (3) are encoded in the form of vivid sensations and images that cannot be accessed by linguistic means alone, (4) are difficult to assimilate and integrate because they are stored differently and are dissociated from conscious awareness and voluntary control, and (5) often remain fixed in their original form and unaltered by the passage of time.

Similarly, Vardi and colleagues (1994) found the presence of more primary sensory stimuli (visual, auditory, kinesthetic) contained in the traumatic memories of rape and incest victims than in their nontraumatic memories. They also reported that the traumatic memories of incest victims were significantly more fragmentary and less continuous than those of rape victims.

The age of the victim at the time of the trauma also appears to influence the manner in which the traumatic memories are encoded. Bruner (1973) noted that a child's earliest memories are encoded in the sensorimotor system, that visual representation becomes dominant between the ages of 2 and 7, and that linguistic representation develops much more slowly and is not fully integrated with the kinesthetic and visual modes until adolescence—all of which appears consistent with Piaget's theory of the stages of cognitive development in children.

TYPE I VS. TYPE II TRAUMA

As described by Terr (1991), type I traumas are unexpected, isolated traumatic events of limited duration (e.g., a single incident of rape, natural disasters, car accidents, industrial accidents, sniper shootings), from which quick recovery is more likely. By contrast, type II traumas are more long-standing in nature and generally involve a series of expected, repeated traumatic events (e.g., ongoing childhood sexual or physical abuse) that lead to a negatively altered schematic view of self and others, accompanied by intense feelings of guilt, shame, worthlessness, helplessness, and hopelessness. Type II traumas such as CSA frequently develop into a more complex and chronic PTSD response associated with other psychiatric conditions, including higher rates of substance abuse, eating disorders, mood disorders, chronic relationship difficulties, and long-standing characterological disturbances evidenced by emotional lability, self-abusive behaviors, and chronic suicidality. Recovery from type II traumas generally takes much longer.

INFORMATION-PROCESSING MODELS OF PTSD

As the conceptualization of PTSD has developed in recent years, information-processing models that emphasize the role of "emotional networks" have gained considerable support as explanations of PTSD symptomatology. While PTSD is considered to be a normal and common response to severe trauma, there appears to be widespread agreement among information-processing theorists that (1) perceptions of the traumatic event can contribute to the development of chronic PTSD, (2) PTSD results not from traumatic events alone but from inadequate emotional processing of the traumas, and (3) PTSD symptoms significantly decrease once adequate or successful emotional processing has occurred (Foa and Kozak 1986, Smucker et al. 1995). Accordingly, it is the victim's response to trauma—and not the traumatic events themselves—that produces a PTSD syndrome. Similarly, it is the individual's response to his/her PTSD symptomatology that determines the course of recovery (Smucker 1997). Consensus, however, has not been reached on what exactly constitutes adequate emotional processing of traumatic material, or on what specific interventions can best facilitate such processing.

INDICATORS OF EMOTIONAL PROCESSING

A number of theorists have recently elaborated on the nature of emotional processing and how it may be impeded or facilitated. In his theory of emotional processing of fear, Rachman

(1980) proposed that successful emotional processing could "be gauged from the person's ability to talk about, see, listen to, or be reminded of the emotional events without experiencing distress or disruptions" (pp. 51–52). Expanding on Piaget's theory of adaptation, Horowitz (1986) hypothesized that the processing of traumatic material is complete once the cognitive schemata have been altered to incorporate and integrate the new information. Until such processing occurs, he noted, a "completion tendency" causes unintegrated material (e.g., recurring flashbacks and nightmares) to emerge repetitively. Successful emotional processing of traumatic events is often frequently delayed or prevented by means of denial, numbing, amnesia, or other dissociative strategies, which, according to Horowitz, are defense maneuvers designed to protect victims from information overload and the affective distress associated with their traumatization. Thus, the oscillation between PTSD intrusions and denial/numbing responses is viewed as a naturally occurring feature prior to a complete integration of the traumatic material.

According to Lang's (1979, 1986) theory of emotional processing, fear-inducing memories are encoded in a neural "network" consisting of stimuli, responses, and the subjective meaning assigned to the stimulus and response data. Lang contended that vivid response imagery and affective involvement must be present in both accessing and altering a fear memory.

Foa and Kozak (1986), who expanded Lang's theory by placing greater emphasis on the cognitive meaning of the trauma, defined emotional processing as "the modification of memory structures that underlie emotions" (p. 20). From their work with adult rape victims, they concluded that recovery from PTSD requires activation of the entire "fear network"—along with the associated affect—and incorporation of corrective information that is incompatible with traumatic elements of the fear structure. Foa and Kozak proposed that prolonged exposure, which confronts the fear stimuli via imaginal flooding, is useful for both activating the fear memory and providing an opportunity for corrective information to be integrated. As such, activation of the fear memory, combined with the absence of objective danger, is thought to provide incompatible information resulting in a physiological habituation to the fear stimuli, which changes the meaning of the fear memory and leads to a modification of the fear structure and reduction of PTSD symptoms. Prolonged imaginal exposure has yielded positive results in alleviating PTSD symptomatology with adult rape victims suffering from type I traumas (Rothbaum and Foa 1992).

More recently, Smucker and colleagues (1995) noted that "the meanings which victims ascribe to their childhood sexual traumas greatly exceed the relationship between perceived danger and physiological reactivity" (p. 7). Contending that exposure to the fear memory alone may not, by itself, provide corrective information regarding abuse-related beliefs and schemas for CSA victims, Smucker and colleagues expanded the definition of "meaning elements" to simultaneously account for the PTSD symptoms (e.g., recurring flashbacks), the abuse-related attributions/beliefs, and the deeply seated traumagenic schemas. While emphasizing the need for imaginal exposure to be a component of treatment with adult CSA survivors, the authors proposed actively modifying the intrusive abuse imagery as well (i.e., changing the victimization imagery to mastery/coping imagery), as a means of providing corrective information both for eliminating the PTSD intrusive imagery and for confronting the underlying traumagenic schemas.

TRANSFORMING TRAUMA INTO WORDS: A CRITICAL COMPONENT OF HEALING

A number of writers have emphasized the need for traumatized individuals to put their experiences into words as a crucial feature of their healing and recovery. Shakespeare was apparently aware of this phenomenon, as noted in the following quote from *Macbeth*: "Give sorrow words; the grief that does not speak whispers the o'er-fraught heart and bids it break" (IV: iii, 209). Similarly, Bettelheim (1984) concluded, "What cannot be talked about can also not be put to rest; and if it is not, the wounds continue to fester" (p. 166). Van der Kolk and van der Hart (1991) have likewise argued that the visual, auditory, and kinesthetic sensations of recurring traumatic memories must be transformed into language before they can be adequately processed and integrated into existing mental schemas. Meichenbaum (1994) elaborated on how the use of language to develop a narrative of the traumatic experience is an essential feature in recovery:

> Accounts are people's story-like construction of events. Victims/survivors who provide well-developed accounts are more likely to develop a perspective on events, become more hopeful about the future, and develop closure regarding stressors. When people fail to talk about a traumatic experience they tend to live with it, dream about it, and ruminate about it, in an unresolved manner. This repetitive or recurrent process provokes higher arousal levels, higher depression and illness rates. By putting these images and their accompanying emotions into language, they become more organized, understood and resolved. [p. 448]

There is some empirical evidence that supports the critical role that talking about one's traumas plays in the healing and recovery process. Harvey and colleagues (1991) used "account-making" (story-like constructions of the traumatic events that include explanations, descriptions, memories, and emotional reactions) and "confiding" (sharing one's account of the traumatic events with an empathic listener) to help trauma survivors more effectively cope with their sexual assault and attain a better overall adjustment. Silver and colleagues (1983) reported that when adult incest survivors were able not only to relate but also to "find meaning in their misfortune," they reported significantly less psychological distress and improved self-esteem, and achieved a better social adaptation and greater resolution of their trauma. Similarly, Pennebaker (1993) reported positive results with trauma victims (e.g., Holocaust survivors) who were able to write or talk about their experiences. Subjects reported lowered autonomic nervous system activity, fewer physician visits, improvement in their long-term immune functioning, and better overall adjustment.

In his review of the trauma literature, Meichenbaum (1994) concluded that writing and talking about traumatic events can have the following benefits:

1. facilitate the expression and labeling of feelings;
2. make the thoughts and feelings about the event more organized (i.e., since language is both more structured and social, talking and writing forces one's thoughts to be implicitly more integrated, less fragmented, leading to a more coherent explanation and an increased likelihood of accepting unchangeable aspects of the situation);
3. influence the accessibility of the thoughts and feelings (i.e., not being as preoccupied as a result of putting their stories into words) and solicit feedback from others;
4. foster some insight and reframing about their predicament and reach some degree of acceptance about themselves and closure about their situation;
5. provide an opportunity to explore the meaning of events and reconsider their reactions; draw connections between past events and present circumstances;
6. foster new perspectives and creative problem solving (p. 449).

2

A Conceptual Overview

The concurrent presence of chronic posttraumatic stress symptoms, maladaptive trauma-related beliefs and schemas in survivors of childhood trauma suggests the need for a treatment approach that simultaneously addresses these different levels of pathology. Thus, imagery rescripting and reprocessing therapy (IRRT) was developed as an expanded information-processing, schema-focused model in which the recurring traumatic memories are conceptualized both within a PTSD framework and as part of the individual's core schemata. Although the primary emphasis in this book is on treating adult survivors of childhood sexual abuse, this treatment intervention is applicable to any childhood trauma (including physical or emotional abuse) manifested in adult PTSD. An extension of Beck's cognitive therapy model (Beck 1976, Beck et al. 1979) and Foa's extinction model (Foa and Kozak 1986), the procedure employs both imagery and verbal interventions to activate the entire fear memory (i.e., the visual, affective, sensory, and cognitive components), as well as to identify, challenge, and modify the recurring traumatic imagery along with associated beliefs and schemas. The use of imagery enables the traumagenic schemas (e.g., schemas of powerlessness, unlovability, mistrust, abandonment) to be visually activated through the eyes of the traumatized child, and challenged, modified, and reprocessed through the eyes of the empowered adult.

The combination of imaginal exposure, mastery imagery, and self-nurturing imagery, along with verbal/linguistic processing and schema-modification, is designed to go beyond extinction models not only in facilitating recovery from PTSD, but also in altering recurring traumatic images, creating more adaptive schemas, and enhancing one's capacity for self-nurturance—all of which are deemed essential for adequate emotional processing to occur.

While rooted in cognitive theories of emotional processing, IRRT also draws on aspects of attachment theory and object relations theory. Imagery interventions serve not only to reduce primary sensory stimuli and PTSD symptoms (e.g., recurring visual flashbacks), challenge maladaptive trauma-related beliefs, and promote schema shifts, but also to establish a therapeutic secure base, foster introject change (i.e., confront and replace hostile introjects with self-soothing introjects), and develop more effective self-calming and self-nurturing strategies. An important distinction is noted between primary cognitive processing and secondary cognitive processing (Smucker 1997). The skillful interweaving of these two levels of processing is viewed as crucial in the successful reworking of childhood trauma.

CLINICAL APPLICATIONS OF IMAGERY: AN HISTORICAL OVERVIEW

The application of imagery within a therapeutic context has its roots in the latter part of the nineteenth century in Europe. Pierre Janet (1898, 1919) employed a procedure that he called "imagery substitution" (replacing one image with another) with hysterical patients. In the 1890s, Freud noted the spontaneous images and imagined scenes that his patients sometimes experienced and perceived "with all the vividness of reality" (Breuer and Freud, 1895/1955, p. 53). It appears that prior to 1900, Freud's clinical application of imagery interventions was quite extensive. One technique he employed involved pressing his hand on the patient's head and instructing the patient to observe the images that emerged as he relaxed the pressure. Freud reported that patients spontaneously started to see in rapid succession various scenes related to their central conflict. Eventually, however, Freud came to regard imagery as a form of resistance that stood in the way of free association and defended the patient against unacceptable impulses. Remarking that his therapy consisted of "wiping away these pictures" (Kosbab 1974, p. 284), Freud gravitated toward verbal methods, in particular free association and dream interpretation. Freud's influence thus resulted in viewing imagery as a more primitive primary process (primarily iconic and illogical in nature) associated with regressive features, which he downplayed in favor of a more rational secondary process (the verbal content of the patient's cognitions relating to more reality-based, directed, logical thought) (Moore and Fine 1990).

Carl Jung (1960), on the other hand, viewed mental imagery as a creative process of the psyche to be employed for attaining greater individual, interpersonal, and spiritual integration. Jung believed in mind–body unity as a life process and suggested that imagery is a means of perceiving and experiencing this life process: "The psyche consists essentially of images. It is a series of images in the truest sense, not an accidental juxtaposition or sequence but a structure that is throughout full of meaning and purpose; it is a 'picturing' of vital activities" (p. 325).

Jung further believed that our unconscious is in a state of constant dreaming, but since our attention is primarily focused on the external, we become aware of our imaginal world only if we specifically focus on it. Much of Jung's own clinical work with patients focused on their images and actively using their creative imagination to help them address their neurotic conflicts. From his own clinical work, Jung (1976) observed, "When you concentrate on a mental picture, it begins to stir, and the image becomes enriched by details. It moves and develops... and so when we concentrate on our inner pictures, our unconscious will produce a series of images which makes a complete story" (p. 172).

Jung coined the term *active imagination* to denote that images have a life of their own and the symbolic events develop according to their own logic, if our conscious reasoning does not interfere. Jung further believed that this active imagination process was superior to dreams in "defeating" the unconscious and quickening maturation.

Albert Binet (1922), though known primarily for his study of the relationship of intelligence to various mental facilities, also recognized the clinical importance of images on an individual's affective state. Binet encouraged patients to converse with their visual images in an introspective state (called "provoked introspection"), a technique that he labeled the "dialogue method."

IMAGERY APPLICATIONS WITHIN A COGNITIVE-BEHAVIORAL CONTEXT

The use of imagery as a primary therapeutic agent in fostering emotional processing of traumatic events has been emphasized by a number of cognitive-oriented clinicians and theorists.* According to van der Kolk and van der Hart (1991), traumatic memories (regardless of the victim's age) and their associated meanings are generally encoded as vivid images and sensations and are not accessible through linguistic retrieval alone. This corroborates the claims of many survivors

---

*See Beck and colleagues (1985) and Edwards (1990) for a review of clinical applications of imagery in cognitive therapy.

of childhood trauma who report much difficulty in linguistically accessing and processing their traumatic childhood memories, and has implications for the use of imagery in treating this population. As noted by Staton (1990), in the absence of corrective imagery, traumatic imagery may be retained no matter how much "talk" occurs. Similarly, Beck and associates (1990) concluded:

> Simply talking about a traumatic event may give intellectual insight about why the patient has a negative self-image, but it does not actually change the image. In order to modify the image, it is necessary to go back in time, as it were, and recreate the situation. When the interactions are brought to life, the misconstruction is activated—along with the affect—and cognitive restructuring can occur. [p. 92]

Other writers have elaborated further on the process of modifying traumatic imagery as a means of reframing the traumatic event and transforming its meaning (e.g., Peterson et al. 1991, Smucker and Niederee 1995). Indeed, if the cognitive/affective disturbance associated with traumatic childhood memories (e.g., recurring flashbacks, repetitive nightmares) is embedded in the traumatic imagery itself, it follows that directly challenging and modifying the distressing imagery becomes a potent means of providing corrective information and facilitating the processing of the traumatic material.

ATTACHMENT THEORY AND ITS RELEVANCE

According to attachment theory, psychotherapy is a process of reappraising and reworking inadequate, dysfunctional, outdated schematic models of the self and attachment figures (Bowlby 1988). A central task of the therapist is providing a reliable and secure base from which patients may begin the arduous task of exploring and reworking their internal working models (Bretherton 1987). Similarly, in IRRT a primary task of the therapist is providing a secure base or safety zone that serves as a therapeutic anchor, within which the patient's unresolved traumatic material can be reexperienced, rescripted, and reprocessed. The therapist facilitates cognitive and affective shifts back and forth in the therapy session from the secure therapeutic base to the anxiety-provoking imagery of the patient's traumatic material. This procedure is somewhat analogous to Wolpe's (1958) systematic desensitization therapy, which involves facilitating repeated patient shifts from a state of relaxation to graded exposure to phobic stimuli, followed by a return to the relaxed state, and so on until the individual is able to remain in a relatively relaxed state during exposure to the phobic stimuli.

OBJECT RELATIONS THEORY AND THE ROLE OF INTROJECTS

Consistent with a basic therapeutic tenet from object relations theory (Ford et al. 1997, Henry et al. 1990), an eventual goal of IRRT with victims of childhood trauma is for them to develop a positive therapist introject that competes with, and eventually replaces, their hostile introjects (which are frequently identified as negative parental introjects). This new therapist introject is thought to create a basis for the development of more adaptive schemata. When activated or summoned up by the patient, this internal cognitive representation of the therapist, which is primarily visual and auditory in nature, may have a calming/soothing effect on the patient's mood, especially during times of emotional distress. (For some distressed patients, activating a positive image of the therapist, or hearing the therapist's soothing voice, can serve as a major affective tranquilizer.) The eventual therapeutic goal is for this positive therapist introject to become integrated into the patient's schematic internal representation of self, such that trauma victims can develop an enhanced capacity to self-calm and self-soothe, especially when feeling upset.

Although the term *introject* has traditionally been used within a psychodynamic context, it may also be viewed as a useful cognitive construct to denote the way in which an individual has schematically internalized (both cognitively and behaviorally) the treatment received by early caregivers, which is reflected in how the individual views and treats him- or herself today. While treatment by early caregivers is viewed as critical to the process of introject formation, the nature and content of introjects are subject to further development and modification across the life span (Henry et al. 1990).

PRIMARY VS. SECONDARY COGNITIVE PROCESSING

An important distinction is noted between primary cognitive processing and secondary cognitive processing, which are refinements of the psychoanalytic terms *primary process* and *secondary process* that Freud coined to reflect two fundamentally different modes of cognitive functioning. In short, Freud viewed the primary process as the earliest, most primitive and illogical form of mentation that is primarily iconic in nature, lacking in temporal dimension, and reflected in such mental activities as daydreams, fantasies, dreams, and slips of the tongue phenomena. By contrast, Freud viewed the secondary process as governed by more reality-based, logical thought and exemplified by delayed gratification and problem-solving activities (Moore and Fine 1990).

In IRRT, the activation of imagery (e.g., traumatic imagery) is viewed as a primary cognitive process (i.e., a mental activity that is primarily visual and auditory in nature). By contrast, secondary cognitive processing refers to the activation of the individual's verbal cognitions (e.g., through talking or writing) as a means of linguistically processing thoughts and feelings about an event.

In IRRT processing traumatic material at both primary and secondary levels is considered essential for successful emotional processing to occur. This is in contrast to some applications of cognitive therapy, for example cognitive processing therapy (Resick and Schnicke 1993), that promote processing traumatic cognitive material at a secondary (verbal) level only. Primary cognitive processing is at work during all imagery phases of exposure and rescripting (i.e., whenever imagery of any kind is activated), although secondary cognitive processing is usually occurring simultaneously during imagery activation. Verbalizing aloud activated traumatic images is, in itself, a form of secondary cognitive processing, as it involves applying words to images. From time to time, throughout each imagery session, the patient and therapist "freeze" the imagery (or put the imagery "on pause") and linguistically process thoughts and feelings that the patient is experiencing about the imagery. The therapist and patient typically go back and forth during an imagery session from primary cognitive processing (i.e., developing and experiencing the imagery) to secondary cognitive processing (i.e., verbalizing thoughts and feelings about the imagery as well as its idiosyncratic meaning). The skillful interweaving of these two levels of cognitive processing is viewed as crucial to the successful emotional processing of traumatic material during imagery sessions.

At the end of each imagery session, patients are also asked to verbalize their thoughts and feelings about the session (i.e., to linguistically process primary cognitive material at a secondary level). This primary and secondary cognitive processing is continued beyond the therapy session as part of the patient's homework, which involves listening daily to an audiotape of the imagery session just completed and recording reactions in a journal.

GOALS OF IRRT

The goals of IRRT are as follows:

1. decrease physiological arousal;
2. eliminate intrusive posttraumatic stress symptoms (e.g., recurring flashbacks, repetitive nightmares);
3. replace victimization imagery with mastery/coping imagery;
4. modify maladaptive, trauma-related cognitions and schemas;
5. develop an enhanced capacity to self-soothe and self-nurture, especially during times of emotional distress;
6. develop more effective coping strategies for dealing with daily life stressors;
7. develop a healthy therapeutic alliance that may ultimately be used to replace the patient's hostile introjects with positive therapist introjects;
8. find positive existential meaning in the traumatic experiences;
9. ultimately view oneself as a survivor and a thriver instead of as a victim.

Altering memories, planting memories, retrieving memory fragments, or reconstructing vague or absent memories for conjectured abuse experiences are *not* goals of IRRT. Only specific trauma-related images/memories that the patient is currently reporting are addressed. The contents of specific traumatic memories are essentially treated as distressing cognitions to be identified, examined, and, when applicable, replaced with more adaptable cognitions/images.

PART II

IMAGERY RESCRIPTING AND REPROCESSING THERAPY

3
Pretreatment Evaluation

Before a patient is accepted for IRRT, a pretreatment evaluation is conducted primarily for the purpose of information gathering, diagnostic assessment, and treatment planning. Information is gathered about the patient's current life situation, family history, history of traumatic and victimization experiences, current psychological adjustment, medical history, alcohol and drug use, depression, and severity of posttraumatic stress symptoms. Much of the pretreatment evaluation focuses on the immediate presenting problems, the degree to which they interfere with daily functioning, the response of the patient's social milieu (e.g., family, friends, employer, co-workers), and how the patient has attempted to cope with the symptoms. Specific questions are asked about the presence, frequency, and intensity of intrusive traumatic recollections, dissociative flashbacks, and repetitive nightmares, which are recorded on the Traumatic Flashback Incident Record (Appendix E). It is important to be sensitive to the emotional state of the patient while probing these areas.

In an attempt to cope with their trauma-related PTSD symptoms, some victims may engage in significant cognitive avoidance behaviors that temporarily reduce the degree of related affective distress, but also significantly reduce their overall level of adaptive functioning. These individuals may avoid going into public places or engaging in situations that could trigger trauma-related memories, anxiety, or fear. Therefore, the clinician needs to conduct a careful behavioral assessment of their daily activities to ascertain the degree of maladaptive avoidance behaviors that may be present.

Clinical assessment measures are also given that can be readministered at the termination of treatment and at followup. The specific preevaluation forms and assessment measures may vary in accordance with the clinician's preferences. Measures frequently used with this population include the following: Beck Depression Inventory (BDI; Beck et al. 1961), Childhood Incest Questionnaire (Edwards and Donaldson 1989), Civilian Version of the Mississippi PTSD Scale (Vreven et al. 1995), Dissociative Experiences Scale (DES; Bernstein and Putnam 1986), Impact of Events Scale–Revised (IES-R; Weiss and Marmar 1996), Incest History Questionnaire (Courtois 1996), Peritraumatic Dissociative Experiences Questionnaire (PDEQ; Marmar et al. 1996), Posttraumatic Stress Diagnostic Scale (PDS; Foa 1995), Revised Mississippi Scale (RCMS; Norris and Perilla 1996), Structured Clinical Interview for *DSM-IV* (SCID I and II; Spitzer et al. 1989), State-Trait Anxiety Inventory (STAI; Spielberger et al. 1970, Spielberger 1982), Trauma Symptom Checklist-40 (TSC-40; Elliott and Briere 1992), Trauma Symptom Inventory (TSI; Briere 1995), TSI Belief Scale–Revision L (Pearlman 1996), and World Assumption Scale (Janoff-Bulman 1996). See Carlson (1996) and Stamm (1996) for a compendium of PTSD clinical assessment measures.

RECOMMENDED INCLUSION CRITERIA

In general, IRRT is likely to be appropriate if the patient recalls or experiences at least one traumatic episode via repeated involuntary, intrusive recollections, recurring visual flashbacks, and/or repetitive nightmares. It is important that the individual remember most or all of the traumatic event(s).

RECOMMENDED EXCLUSION CRITERIA

Although the decision of whether to use IRRT lies ultimately with the clinician (in collaboration with the patient), situations in which it typically is not indicated include:

- Current involvement in a highly abusive relationship (in such instances, therapy should first focus on helping patients extricate themselves from the abuse situation);
- A diagnosis of schizophrenia, severe dissociative identity disorder, or acute psychosis;
- Active involvement in substance or alcohol abuse (in such instances, therapy should first focus on helping the patient confront, and abstain from, the addictive behaviors);
- The presence of overwhelming, day-to-day stressors;
- The presence of vague or incomplete traumatic memories;
- The absence of traumatic visual memories.

CONCOMITANT USE OF MEDICATION

It is not uncommon for patients treated with IRRT to be simultaneously taking mood-stabilizing medications. Indeed, if the patient's affective instability is such that s/he is unable to implement and benefit from this treatment without the aid of psychiatric medication, it may be advisable to refer the patient to a psychiatrist for a psychopharmacological evaluation before beginning with the imagery sessions.

INTRODUCING IRRT TO THE PATIENT

If, by the end of the pretreatment evaluation session, the appropriateness of IRRT is established, the following brief description of the treatment may be offered to the patient:

> This treatment is designed to help you overcome and master your traumatic memories and leave you feeling more empowered and in control of your life. At the beginning of the next session, I will describe the therapy to you in detail.

Any questions, concerns, or fears the patient may have are addressed in a succinct manner. It is generally best *not* to describe the treatment in more detail at this point. If the patient persists with additional questions about what the procedure involves, the therapist may repeat in a calm and reassuring manner:

> This procedure will help you to process your painful memories and get on with your life in a more meaningful way. It's probably best, however, that we wait until next session to address any further questions you might still have about the treatment.

Before the pretreatment evaluation session is ended, the therapist takes a few minutes to teach the patient a brief focused-breathing exercise, similar to what is typically used with patients suffering from panic attacks (Clark 1986). It is important that patients be able to take something positive with them from this initial session, and helping them to get into a more relaxed state via a breathing exercise is often a very efficient and effective means of accomplishing this. (Beginning and ending subsequent sessions with such a breathing exercise has also been found to be useful for many patients.)

4

Exposure, Rescripting, and Self-Nurturing Imagery

SESSION 1: BEGINNING TREATMENT

Assess general mood
Record presence/frequency of recurring flashbacks and nightmares on the Traumatic Flashback Incident Record
Present treatment rationale
Introduce subjective units of distress (SUDs)
Facilitate imaginal exposure: reexperiencing the traumatic scene
Facilitate mastery imagery: rescripting the traumatic scene
Facilitate adult-nurturing-child imagery
Administer the Post-Imagery Questionnaire-A (PIQ-A)
Process and debrief
Assess self-calming and self-soothing abilities
Contract for safety
Assign homework

Allow two hours for session 1. The first few minutes are spent reviewing the patient's general mood and any thoughts, feelings, questions, or fears about the pretreatment evaluation or the treatment itself. The therapist should show sensitivity while responding succinctly to any concerns the patient might express. Above all, the therapist's tone of voice should be calm, gentle, and confident, and should convey a sense of reassurance to the patient.

The therapist then inquires about the presence and frequency of traumatic intrusive memories, recurring flashbacks, and repetitive nightmares that the patient has experienced since the evaluation and records this information on the Traumatic Flashback Incident Record (Appendix E).

Presenting the Treatment Rationale

It is important that patients be adequately educated about the nature of their symptoms and about how posttraumatic stress symptoms result from inadequate emotional processing of traumatic events. Patients should be told that this treatment is designed to help them emotionally process their painful experiences so that they can move forward with their lives. The therapist presents the rationale for treatment to the patient in the following manner, which may be paraphrased in the therapist's own words:

> When we undergo a trauma, we experience a sense of extreme danger, whether physical, emotional, or both. The natural response to such an event is intense fear, which involves urges to fight, flee, or freeze. These responses are normal, automatic reactions to danger. They can affect our bodies (e.g., heart pounding, sweating), our thoughts (e.g., thinking we are in danger), and our actions (e.g., trying to get away). These intense responses can reoccur years after the trauma if something in our lives triggers memories of the event.
>
> All aspects of your traumatic experience exist in a network of memories. Body sensations, odors, time of day or night, or the place in which the trauma occurred may all become part of this memory. It is like a "fear network" in your mind.
>
> If you think about the traumatic event or see something reminding you of it, you may experience intense feelings of

fear, disgust, guilt, shame, rage, or sorrow—much like what you felt at the time of the trauma. Reexperiencing these feelings causes great distress, which is why most people try to push away these painful memories or ignore them. You may tell yourself, "I should just forget about the whole thing and not let it bother me anymore," or "If I don't think about it, it will eventually go away."

Some people may try to convince you that avoidance is the best way to cope with trauma. Friends, relatives, or even partners may feel uncomfortable hearing about your experience and discourage you from talking about it. Unfortunately, trying to ignore your feelings and fears does not make them go away. Often the traumatic event comes back to haunt you through painful recurring memories, flashbacks, or nightmares because it is "unfinished business."

As you know from your own experience, it is not easy to recover from childhood traumas. How you view yourself, others, and the world in general has been dramatically affected by your trauma. You may find it difficult to believe in yourself or to trust anyone. We are here to help you with this.

The purpose of our work together here is to help you work through, and move beyond, your traumatic memories. We have found that this treatment not only helps people like yourself overcome trauma-related memories, it also helps them to develop a healthier self-image and to move forward with their lives as "thrivers."

The therapist may pause briefly at this point to address any questions the patient might have, after which details of the treatment are described to the patient:

Much of the work we will be doing involves the use of imagery or visualization. The therapy involves asking you to visually recall and reexperience the traumatic images, thoughts, and feelings you experience during a flashback (or nightmare). Initially, I will ask you to visualize the entire memory in imagery as you remember it. Then we will go back over it again and this time change, or rescript, the imagery to create a better outcome for you, one that leaves you feeling more empowered and in control. The aim is to replace your victimization images with mastery images so that you can see and feel yourself responding to your trauma no longer as a victim, but as an empowered individual. This, of course, does not change the traumatic events themselves, but it can change the lingering images, thoughts, feelings, and beliefs that you have about the trauma. Do you have any questions?

A written copy of the above treatment rationale (Appendix A) is given to the patient to take home and refer to, should questions regarding the purpose or treatment rationale arise between sessions. Patients are fully informed of the short-term emotional distress and heightened state of arousal that may occur when traumatic imagery is experienced in the therapy session. This information, however, should be considered within the context of the affective distress that the patient is already experiencing when intrusive, traumatic recollections or flashbacks are activated outside of the therapist's office.

It is important to emphasize that this is not a harsh treatment, that the patient is already being traumatized and retraumatized by the presence of these recurring traumatic images, and that activating the traumatic flashbacks in the session offers an opportunity for the therapist to assist the patient in developing coping strategies to gain control and mastery over these recurring, distressing images. The therapist may also emphasize that reexperiencing painful memories in a therapy session is different from experiencing the actual event, that the trauma is in actuality not occurring, and that the therapist's voice and supportive presence provide a therapeutic anchor throughout the imagery sessions. Finally, patients are encouraged to contact the therapist between sessions if the need arises. (The therapist or a qualified colleague should be available for emergencies on a 24-hour basis.)

Inviting Questions and Validating Patient Concerns

Patients are invited to ask any questions they might have about their traumatic experiences or the therapy itself. Any patient questions, concerns, or fears are generally addressed in a succinct and candid manner. It is crucial that the patient feel listened to, understood, and validated. Because the therapeutic alliance is so critical to effective outcomes with this patient population, it is highly advisable to ask the patients specific questions regarding their current thoughts and feelings about working with the therapist, and any concerns they might have regarding trust. It is normal and natural for trauma victims to feel a strong sense of mistrust toward anyone to whom they will be pouring out their soul, and these feelings need to be heard, normalized, and validated by the therapist.

Introducing Subjective Units of Distress (SUDs)

Following the presentation of the treatment rationale and validation of patient questions or concerns, patients are taught to use a SUDs rating (on a 0 to 100 scale) to indicate the degree of distress or discomfort they feel. This may be explained as follows:

> As part of this treatment, you will be asked to experience memories and scenes that will generate some anxiety and discomfort. From time to time, I will be asking you to monitor and rate the amount of discomfort you are feeling on a scale from 0 to 100. A rating of 100 would indicate that you are feeling extremely upset, the most distressed you have ever felt. A rating of 0 would indicate that you are feeling no discomfort at all. Using this scale, how much discomfort or distress might you be feeling at this moment?

The therapist records on the Therapist Record (Appendix C) the patient's SUDs level at the beginning and end of each imagery phase and at approximately every ten minutes within each imagery phase. The clinician may also ask for SUDs levels at other times during the imagery, provided that it be done purposively and sparingly and not distract from the imagery.

Imaginal Exposure: Reexperiencing the Traumatic Event

This phase of the session includes visual and sensory reliving of the entire traumatic memory. Initially, the patient is asked to visualize and verbalize aloud the entire traumatic experience in the present tense, as if it were occurring at the moment. If the patient reports experiencing a number of different recurring flashbacks or nightmares, each distressing memory is identified, a SUDs level for each memory is elicited, and the patient is asked which memory might best be targeted for initial treatment. The therapist introduces the imaginal exposure phase as follows:

> I am going to ask you to recall the entire traumatic memory. I would encourage you to close your eyes so you won't be distracted. I will be asking you to recall these painful memories as vividly as possible. It is important that you describe the traumatic event in the present tense, as if it were happening now, right here. We will work together on this. If you start to feel too uncomfortable and want to leave the image, I will help you to stay with it and regain a sense of safety. From time to time I'll ask you to rate your level of discomfort on a 0 to 100 scale. Please answer quickly and do not leave the image. Do you have any questions before we start?

Any questions the patient might have are best addressed in a brief and reassuring manner. Abstract, lengthy, or involved questions are preferably deferred until the end of the imagery session. The therapist then continues with the following instructions:

> I'd like you now to close your eyes and visualize the beginning of the traumatic event, and describe in detail what you experience, including thoughts and feelings you have about what is happening. Again it is important that you describe your experience in the present tense, as if it were happening now.

During imaginal exposure, the therapist's role is facilitative rather than directive. The therapist does not intervene other than to ask the patient for details of the traumatic event or to elaborate on thoughts and feelings about what is happening. It is crucial that the entire fear network be activated during imaginal exposure, which includes visual, verbal, affective, sensory, and kinesthetic stimuli.

The imaginal exposure continues until the verbalized account of the entire memory appears to have ended, at which time the therapist asks, "Is there anything more that happens in the imagery?" Once the patient confirms that the traumatic imagery has ended and it is clear that the patient has reexperienced and verbalized the entire traumatic memory, the imaginal exposure phase is brought to a close, and the therapist immediately facilitates a transition to the next phase of imagery. There is no processing or debriefing at this point. Any questions or comments the patient may have should be gently, but firmly, deferred until the end of the session.

Mastery Imagery: Rescripting the Traumatic Imagery

Upon completion of the imaginal exposure phase, the therapist begins the mastery imagery phase as follows:

> I'd like you once again to visualize the beginning of the traumatic scene and describe, in the present, what is happening. This time, however, when you get to a certain point in the imagery, we will change it to a better outcome, and I will help you with this. Are you ready to begin?

Again, any questions the patient may have about the rescripting phase are best deferred until the end of the imagery session. Once the patient has indicated a readiness to begin, the therapist may proceed as follows:

> When you are ready, you may once again visualize the beginning of the traumatic scene and describe in detail what is happening.

Initially, the rescripting phase closely resembles the exposure imagery. However, when the traumatic imagery appears to have reached its zenith—at this point the patient's SUDs should be high—the patient is asked to visualize herself[1] as an adult today entering into the imagery.[2]

The therapist may facilitate this visualization through questions:

> Can you now visualize yourself as an ADULT today entering into the imagery? Can you get a picture of that?
> What happens when you, the ADULT, enter into the imagery?

---

1. Although IRRT has been successfully used in treating both males and females, the feminine pronoun is used here because the vast majority of individuals seeking treatment for the aftereffects of childhood trauma are females.
2. Throughout the mastery and imagery phases, the therapist addresses the ADULT in the second person (as "you") and addresses the CHILD in the third person (as "the CHILD"), so as to strengthen and reinforce the notion that the patient today is an adult and capable of functioning competently as an adult.

EXPOSURE, RESCRIPTING, AND SELF-NURTURING IMAGERY

Does he[3] (the perpetrator) see you?
How does he (the perpetrator) respond to your presence?
What would you, the ADULT, like to do at this point?
Can you see yourself doing that?
And how does he (the perpetrator) respond?
How do you, the ADULT, respond to the perpetrator?
And what is happening now?

The specific purpose of the mastery imagery phase is to replace victimization imagery with coping imagery. Thus, the initial role of the ADULT is to rescript the victimization imagery and produce a better outcome by visually confronting the perpetrator, rescuing the CHILD from the traumatic scene, and providing protection for the CHILD, using whatever means necessary to accomplish this. However, the therapist's role remains primarily facilitative, as the patient is encouraged to decide for herself what coping strategies to use in the mastery imagery.

If the ADULT is unable to visualize herself confronting the perpetrator and rescuing the CHILD, the therapist may eventually ask whether additional support people (e.g., a police officer, therapist, spouse, friend) might be needed to help out. In such instances, however, it is crucial that the patient—*not* the therapist—decide who the support person(s) shall be. Throughout rescripting, it is imperative that the therapist remain nondirective while employing Socratic imagery, as opposed to guided imagery. Socratic imagery is essentially Socratic questioning applied in the context of imagery modification, and derives from the notion that developing one's own mastery/coping imagery is more empowering than to have it suggested, directed, or dictated by the therapist. The therapist must resist any urge to "rescue" the patient

---

3. Although the masculine pronoun is used here, the perpetrator can be male or female, and there can be multiple perpetrators.

from the traumatic imagery, to tell the patient what to do, or to suggest what should be happening in the rescripted imagery.

Developing Adult-Nurturing-Child Imagery

Following successful completion of the master imagery (i.e., after the CHILD has been rescued from the traumatic scene and the perpetrator is out of the picture), the therapist fosters adult-nurturing-child imagery, during which the ADULT interacts directly with the traumatized CHILD. It is critical, however, that the therapist call this phase "Adult–Child imagery," *not* "Adult-Nurturing-Child imagery." Clinical experience has shown that this phase of imagery is less likely to be successful if the client thinks the ADULT should be nurturing the CHILD (as is implied if the therapist refers to this phase as "Adult-Nurturing-Child imagery") and tries to force her ADULT to nurture the CHILD, especially if the ADULT is harboring ill feelings toward the CHILD (e.g., anger, blame, hate). In some instances, the ADULT may first need to express such negative thoughts and feelings to the CHILD directly before any nurturing feelings toward the CHILD can be genuinely felt and expressed.

The therapist facilitates the ADULT–CHILD imagery by asking:

> What would you, the ADULT, like to do or say to the CHILD?
> Can you see yourself doing (or saying) that?
> How does the CHILD respond?
> How do you, the ADULT, respond to the CHILD's response?
> What do you, the ADULT, see when you look directly into the CHILD's eyes?

Quite often at this point the ADULT will begin to hold or hug the CHILD, reassure the CHILD that the abuse or traumatic event will not happen again, and promise not to abandon the CHILD. However, if the ADULT has difficulty nurturing the CHILD, blames the CHILD, or wants to hurt or abandon the CHILD, it is important for the ADULT to express her anger (and other negative feelings) directly to the CHILD from close proximity. These ADULT–CHILD interactions may be facilitated by asking:

> How far away are you, the ADULT, from the CHILD?
> Can you go up close to the CHILD and tell her why you are angry at her/why you want to hurt her/why you want to abandon her?
> Can you look into the CHILD's eyes directly and tell her why you feel she is to blame?[4]
> And how does the CHILD respond?
> When you look directly into the CHILD's eyes, from up close, what do you see?
> How do you, the ADULT, respond to what you see in the CHILD's eyes?
> What would you, the ADULT, now like to do or say to the CHILD?
> Can you visualize yourself doing/saying that?

Generally, as the ADULT moves closer to the CHILD in physical proximity, the ADULT becomes more affected by the CHILD's pain and finds it more difficult to continue blaming, hurting, or abandoning the CHILD. Such intense ADULT–CHILD interactions tend to heighten the patient's overall level of affect and evoke strong feelings toward the

---

4. These questions are not considered a deviation from Socratic imagery. They direct physical proximity, not verbal content, and are used to confront avoidance behaviors in the imagery. In short, the ADULT is not being told what to think or feel, but is being asked to express her thoughts and feelings directly to the CHILD from up close, and to observe the CHILD's reactions from up close.

CHILD that are often empathic, apologetic, or conciliatory in nature.

With more severely disturbed patients, however, such intimate ADULT–CHILD exchanges may activate hostile introjects, or an unlovable schema, during the imagery session, in which strong negative feelings are evoked toward the perceived bad, disgusting, evil, unlovable part of the patient, which the CHILD often seems to represent in the imagery. When this occurs, it provides a unique therapeutic opportunity for the patient to confront her unlovable schema directly via the ADULT–CHILD exchanges and within the context of a supportive, therapeutic relationship. (See Chapter 11 for more on how to confront an activated unlovable schema during an imagery session.)

Once it appears that the ADULT has offered sufficient nurturance to the CHILD and the patient may be ready to end the imagery, the therapist asks:

> Is there anything more that you, the ADULT, would like to do with or say to the CHILD before bringing the imagery to a close?

When the patient indicates a readiness to terminate the imagery session, the therapist concludes:

> You may now let the imagery fade away, and when you are ready you may open your eyes.

Administering the Post-Imagery Questionnaire

After the patient has had several moments to adapt to the completion of the imagery phase, the therapist administers the Post-Imagery Questionnaire-A (PIQ-A) (Appendix B), which involves reading each item aloud to the patient and recording the patient's numerical rating on the line to the left of each item. The PIQ offers immediate and direct patient feedback about the imagery session just experienced and is used to monitor qualitative progress on a session-by-session basis. The PIQ-A is used after all imagery sessions that include imaginal exposure, mastery imagery, and ADULT–CHILD imagery (which, according to the standard format, are sessions 1 to 8), whereas the PIQ-B is used after all imagery sessions that involve only ADULT–CHILD imagery (i.e., session 8 and follow-up).

Processing and Debriefing

After the Post-Imagery Questionnaire has been administered, reactions to the imagery session are discussed and processed together with the patient. To facilitate such processing, the therapist may ask:

> How was that for you?
> How are you feeling now?
> What thoughts and feelings do you have about the imagery session today?
> What did you feel when you, the ADULT, entered the imagery and confronted the perpetrator?
> What were you thinking and feeling when you, the ADULT, first looked directly into the CHILD's eyes?

Above all, the therapist should avoid asking closed-ended or leading questions, such as "Are you feeling better now?"

During the processing and debriefing, the therapist's voice and affective demeanor should be calm, sensitive, reassuring, and attuned to the patient's affective state. If the patient appears noticeably calmer at this point than during the exposure or rescripting phases, the therapist might want to call this to the patient's attention and reinforce the notion that while the processing of traumatic memories is indeed hard work, it is work that nonetheless leads somewhere. It is often useful to frame those pains associated with the emotional processing of traumatic stimuli as "growing pains," contrasted with the "stagnation pains" of not moving forward with one's life in a meaningful way and staying emotionally stuck in one's victimization and traumatization.

Assessing Self-Calming and Self-Soothing Abilities

The therapist inquires about the patient's general ability to self-calm and self-soothe when feeling upset. It is important to emphasize the difference between self-calming strategies that are self-abusive (e.g., cutting or other forms of self-injury) and healthy self-calming strategies that are not abusive (e.g., writing in a journal, working out, relaxing, engaging in a self-nurturing activity, calling a friend or other support person). The therapist and patient then collaboratively explore various self-calming strategies for the patient to experiment with between sessions, especially when feeling upset.

Contracting for Safety

Whether or not there is any previous history of self-abuse or suicidality, it is imperative that the patient contract for safety and agree not to engage in any suicidal, self-harming, or self-abusive behaviors throughout treatment, and to call the therapist between sessions when feeling strong urges to self-abuse or self-harm.

Homework

Homework is presented to the patient as a very important part of treatment, since much of the emotional processing of the traumatic material, as well as the implementation of more effective coping strategies, will be taking place outside of the therapist's office. It is important to emphasize the link between therapy benefits and the amount of effort invested in the homework. Although the homework may seem ambitious to the patient initially, it is important to emphasize that the actual time needed to do the homework will probably be significantly less than the amount of time and energy that the patient is currently expending each day struggling with the trauma-related symptoms and associated pain.

While patients are encouraged to do as much of the homework as they are able—and need to understand that the homework is an essential component of treatment—it is important that they do not feel overly pressured or overwhelmed, or be made to feel that they have failed if they are unable to complete the homework. It is important to allow extra time at the end of the first session to address any questions or concerns that might arise regarding the homework. At the end of each therapy session, a homework assignment sheet is discussed and handed to the patient.

Homework Assignment (Session 1)

After each imagery session, you will be given an audiotape of the imagery session just completed to listen to as part of your daily homework.

I. Process further your reactions to today's imagery session.

1. Listen daily to the audiotape of the entire imagery session (exposure and rescripting).
2. Record SUDs on the Homework Record (Appendix D) both prior to and after listening to the audiotape of the imagery session.
3. Immediately after listening to the audiotaped imagery session, self-administer the PIQ-A and record the PIQ score on the Homework Record.
4. Write in a journal your personal reactions to the audiotape.

5. Record on the Traumatic Flashback Incident Record (Appendix E) any involuntary traumatic flashbacks experienced either while listening or processing reactions to the audiotape, or otherwise.

II. Record efforts to self-calm and self-soothe.

Each time you feel upset and attempt to self-calm, write down the following information:

1. the upsetting situation;
2. the level of distress felt (on a 1 to 10 scale) immediately before and after efforts to self-calm;
3. the upsetting thoughts and images;
4. the specific interventions that you attempted (such as self-soothing imagery, calling a friend, going on a long walk, writing in a journal);
5. how successful each intervention was.

III. Bring homework to next session for review.

At the end of every session, the therapist must be sure that the patient feels safe, is sufficiently in control of his/her emotions, and has a low SUDs level prior to leaving the office.

SESSION 2

Assess general mood and between-session mood shifts
Review homework
    Review reactions to daily audiotape listening
    Review Traumatic Flashback Incident Record data
    Review efficacy of self-calming strategies attempted
Facilitate imaginal exposure, mastery imagery, and ADULT–CHILD imagery
Administer Post-Imagery Questionnaire-A (PIQ-A)
Process and debrief
Review contract for safety (if applicable)
Discuss writing letter to perpetrator
Assign homework

EXPOSURE, RESCRIPTING, AND SELF-NURTURING IMAGERY 57

Allow 90 minutes for session 2. The first few minutes are spent reviewing the patient's general mood, shifts in mood since last session, and reactions to the previous session. The therapist should be sensitive to any anxiety, fearfulness, or affective distress the patient might be manifesting, and encourage the patient to share any thoughts and feelings she might have about the therapy and the therapist. It is important to listen to, understand, clarify, empathize with, and validate whatever concerns the patient might have. Patients often need to feel validated again and again by the therapist, especially early in treatment. Building a solid therapeutic alliance continues to be a *sine qua non* of successful treatment with this clinical population.

The therapist begins by inviting the patient to share general reactions to the homework:

> How did the homework go?
> What were your reactions to the homework?

After briefly processing the patient's general reactions to the homework, the therapist and patient then review in detail the homework together, beginning with the Homework Record and the patient's SUDs data and PIQ scores, which the patient records after each daily listening to the audiotape of the previous session. The therapist will want to look closely at the daily SUDs data and PIQ scores recorded on the Homework Record and determine whether any desensitization may have occurred between the first tape-listening and the most recent one. The therapist also inquires about the presence, frequency, and intensity of flashbacks and nightmares since the previous session and reviews the data recorded on the Traumatic Flashback Incident Record.

The therapist then inquires about the patient's ability since the previous session to self-calm and self-soothe, especially when feeling upset, and reviews the efficacy of the self-calming strategies attempted. The therapist and patient collaboratively explore and decide what specific coping, self-calming strategies the patient will continue to use or experiment with between sessions.

Imaginal Exposure, Mastery Imagery, and ADULT–CHILD Imagery

The next 60 minutes or so involve (1) reexperiencing the traumatic imagery (imaginal exposure), (2) rescripting the traumatic imagery (developing mastery imagery), and (3) developing ADULT–CHILD imagery. Each imagery session follows the same format as in session 1 and begins with the same traumatic memory each time. Throughout all phases of imagery the therapist's role continues to be facilitative rather than directive. The therapist may ask questions about details of the imagery and invite patients to elaborate on their thoughts and feelings about what is happening:

> What is happening now in the imagery?
> And what happens next?

During the imaginal exposure phase, patients sometimes experience more graphic and detailed imagery than they did in the first session, which in turn may heighten their emotional distress. It is crucial that the therapist's voice remain calm and steady throughout. Patients need to feel the therapist's supportive presence throughout the exposure phase, while being allowed to "feel their feelings" and experience their pain without therapist interference. Therapists should not attempt to rescue or protect patients from going through their pain, even though it may at times feel unbearable. (Therapists who have difficulty with this should remember that cognitive and affective avoidance is a detriment to recovery and keeps adult PTSD sufferers stuck in their victimization and pain.)

Frequently, during the rescripting phases of imagery in session 2 (i.e., mastery imagery and the ADULT–CHILD imagery), patients develop imagery that is different from, or goes significantly beyond, that experienced in session 1. For example, it is not uncommon for patients during mastery imagery to feel less fearful of, become more assertive with, or use more physical force with the perpetrator than in the first rescripting session. Patients may also feel more loving and nurturing, or more aggressive or conflicted, toward the CHILD during the ADULT–CHILD imagery phase of session 2 or later sessions.

Regardless of how the imagery develops or is rescripted, the therapist's primary task is to follow the patient through the imagery, while making sure that cognitive and affective avoidance during the imagery is minimized. An example of avoidance behavior during imagery may involve the patient's ADULT being afraid to express anger directly at the perpetrator, or not wanting to look directly into the CHILD's eyes for fear of getting too close to the CHILD's pain and feeling overwhelmed by it. Thus, if during imagery the patient's ADULT begins to verbalize feelings she has toward the perpetrator, or toward the CHILD, in the third person—"I'm really angry at him for hurting the CHILD," or "I feel really bad about all the suffering the CHILD had to go through," or "I feel really angry at the CHILD"—the therapist may ask the ADULT to address the perpetrator or the CHILD directly in the imagery:

> Can you say that to the perpetrator directly?
> Can you go up close to the CHILD, look into the CHILD's eyes, and say that to the CHILD directly?
> Can you tell the CHILD why you are so angry at her?

Although the therapist never tells the ADULT, CHILD, or perpetrator what to say in the imagery, the therapist may confront cognitive or affective avoidance by asking the ADULT to address others in the imagery more directly (e.g., in the second person), move physically closer to them, or engage in more direct eye contact with them. Everything that the ADULT verbalizes about the perpetrator and the CHILD during imagery needs to be said to them directly.

Post-Imagery Processing and Debriefing

Once the patient has completed the exposure, mastery, and ADULT–CHILD imagery phases, and has had several moments to adapt to the completion of the imagery, the therapist administers the PIQ-A, facilitates processing and debriefing of the imagery session, and reviews the safety contract. As reactions to the imagery session are invited, discussed, and processed, the therapist continues to look for opportunities to reinforce the work the patient is doing, offer reassurance, and point out specific areas of progress that the patient appears to be making in the imagery. The safety contract is reviewed and reinforced, and the patient is reminded to telephone the therapist between sessions if strong urges to self-abuse or self-harm arise.

Writing a Letter to the Perpetrator

The therapist then introduces the idea of writing a letter to the perpetrator, in which patients are asked to express their thoughts and feelings about their trauma to the perpetrator directly. (If the patient is unable or unwilling to write a letter to the perpetrator, the therapist may suggest writing a letter to another individual toward whom the patient experiences strong emotional reactions, for example, her mother or grandmother.) The rationale behind writing such a letter may be explained as follows:

Many trauma survivors find it useful to write a letter to the perpetrator in which they express their thoughts and feelings about their experience directly to the perpetrator, and then discuss the letter at the next session. Writing such a letter can help survivors verbally process and work through their painful memories and emotions.

How would you feel about writing such a letter this week as a homework assignment? In our next session you would have the opportunity to read your letter and discuss your thoughts and feelings about it.

The therapist allows sufficient time to discuss reactions to the assignment and makes sure the patient understands that the letter is *not* to be sent. (Even if the patient has written a similar letter in the past, considerable benefit may be derived from writing and emotionally processing another such letter as part of the current treatment.)

Homework Assignment (Session 2)

I. Process further your reactions to today's imagery session.
  1. Listen daily to the audiotape of the entire imagery session (exposure and rescripting).
  2. Record your SUDs on the Homework Record both prior to and after listening to the audiotaped imagery session.
  3. Fill out the PIQ-A and record the PIQ score on the Homework Record immediately after listening to the audiotaped imagery session.
  4. Write out your personal reactions to the audiotaped imagery session in a journal.
  5. Record on the Traumatic Flashback Incident Record any recurring flashbacks or nightmares experienced between sessions.

II. Document efforts to self-calm and self-soothe.

  Each time you feel upset and attempt to self-calm, write down the following information:
  1. the upsetting situation;

2. the level of distress felt (on a 1 to 10 scale) immediately before and after efforts to self-calm;
3. the upsetting thoughts and images;
4. the specific interventions that you attempted (such as self-calming imagery, calling a friend, going on a long walk, working out);
5. how successful each intervention was.

III. Write a letter to the perpetrator.

Write a letter addressed to the perpetrator, in which you express your thoughts and feelings about your experience directly to the perpetrator. Do *not* send the letter. Bring the letter to the next session for processing.

IV. Bring homework to next session for review.

SESSION 3

Assess general mood and between-session mood shifts
Review homework
 Discuss letter to perpetrator
 Review reactions to daily audiotape listening
 Review Traumatic Flashback Incident Record data
 Review efficacy of self-calming strategies attempted
Facilitate imaginal exposure, mastery imagery, and ADULT–CHILD imagery
Administer Post-Imagery Questionnaire-A (PIQ-A)
Process and debrief
Discuss writing out entire traumatic memory
Assign homework
Review contract for safety (if applicable)

Allow two hours for session 3. The first 30 minutes or so are spent reviewing the patient's general mood, shifts in mood since the last session, reactions to the previous session, and homework. The patient is encouraged to read aloud and discuss the letter addressed to the perpetrator. (It may be useful at this point to discuss with the patient the possibility of incorporating information from the letter into the imagery later in the session.) Once the letter to the perpetrator has been read and adequately processed, the therapist and patient together review in detail the remainder of the homework, beginning with the Homework Record. The patient's SUDs data and PIQ scores are compared and contrasted with these data from the previous session to determine if, and how much, across-session or between-session desensitization may be occurring. The therapist also inquires about the presence, frequency, and intensity of flashbacks and nightmares since last session, reviews the data recorded on the Traumatic Flashback Incident Record, and compares these data with those of the previous session to ascertain whether the frequency and intensity of the patient's traumatic recollections are diminishing.

The therapist again inquires about the patient's ability since last session to self-calm and self-soothe, especially when feeling upset, and reviews the efficacy of the self-calming strategies that the patient has attempted. The therapist and patient further explore and decide collaboratively what specific coping, self-calming/self-soothing strategies the patient will continue to use or experiment with between sessions.

In the next 60 minutes or so, the patient reexperiences the traumatic imagery (imaginal exposure), rescripts the traumatic imagery (develops mastery imagery), and develops ADULT–CHILD imagery. Each phase of imagery follows the same format as in session 1 and begins with the same traumatic memory; The therapist's approach remains primarily facilitative and nondirective.

Once the patient has completed the exposure, mastery, and ADULT–CHILD imagery phases, and has had several moments to adapt to the completion of the imagery, the therapist administers the PIQ-A, facilitates processing and debriefing of the imagery session, reviews the safety contract (if applicable), and assigns homework.

Writing Out the Entire Flashback

The therapist introduces the idea of the patient writing out the entire traumatic memory for homework, as a means of (1) more fully activating and integrating all elements of the traumatic experience (i.e., visual, auditory, affective, kinesthetic, and linguistic), (2) enhancing emotional processing of the trauma at a linguistic level, and (3) removing the grip of terror and horror of the abuse experience. The rationale may be explained to the patient as follows:

> Many victims of childhood trauma have found it useful to write down every detail of the entire traumatic memory, from beginning to end. While it is normal to feel some initial fear and anxiety at the thought of writing out an entire flashback, survivors find that this assignment does help them get through the pain and move beyond the past. Transforming the visual, emotional, and physical sensations of traumatic memories into written language helps to remove the grip of terror and horror of the trauma and paves the way for healing to occur.
>
> How would you feel about writing out the entire flashback, including your thoughts and feelings about the event, as part of your homework assignment?

The therapist allows sufficient time to discuss the patient's reactions to the assignment.

Homework Assignment (Session 3)

I. Process further your reactions to today's imagery session.
   1. Listen daily to the audiotape of the entire imagery session (exposure and rescripting).
   2. Record your SUDs on the Homework Record both prior to and after listening to the audiotaped imagery session.
   3. Fill out the PIQ-A and record the PIQ score on the Homework Record immediately after listening to the audiotaped imagery session.

4. Write out your personal reactions to the audiotaped imagery session in a journal.
5. Record on the Traumatic Flashback Incident Record any recurring flashbacks or nightmares experienced between sessions.

II. Document efforts to self-calm and self-soothe.

Each time you feel upset and attempt to self-calm, write down the following information:

1. the upsetting situation;
2. the level of distress felt (on a 1 to 10 scale) immediately before and after efforts to self-calm;
3. the upsetting thoughts and images;
4. the specific interventions that you attempted (such as self-calming imagery, calling a friend, going on a long walk, working out);
5. how successful each intervention was.

III. Write out details of entire traumatic memory.

1. Write out as many details of the actual event as you remember, from beginning to end.
2. As you are writing a description of the event itself (of what actually happened), include:
   a. thoughts and feelings you may have experienced at the time of the trauma, and
   b. reactions you may have today while writing the description.

IV. Bring homework to next session for review.

SESSION 4

Assess general mood and between-session mood shifts
Review homework
    Review reactions to daily audiotape listening
    Review Traumatic Flashback Incident Record data
    Process reactions to writing out entire traumatic memory

Review efficacy of self-calming strategies attempted
Facilitate imaginal exposure, mastery imagery, and ADULT–CHILD Imagery
Administer Post-Imagery Questionnaire-A (PIQ-A)
Process and debrief
Review contract for safety (if applicable)
Discuss writing a follow-up letter
Assign homework

Allow 90 minutes for session 4. The first few minutes of the session are spent reviewing the patient's general mood, shifts in mood since last session, and reactions to the previous session. The therapist and patient then review in detail the homework, beginning with the Homework Record. Close attention is paid to the patient's SUDs data and PIQ scores as a means of monitoring the patient's ongoing progress, and these data are compared with those of previous sessions. Similarly, the therapist inquires about the presence, frequency, and intensity of flashbacks and nightmares since last session, and compares the data recorded on the Traumatic Flashback Incident Record with data from earlier sessions. The patient's reactions to writing out the entire traumatic memory are examined and processed.

The therapist again inquires about the patient's ability between sessions to self-calm and self-soothe when feeling upset, and reviews the efficacy of the self-calming strategies that the patient has attempted. Comparisons may be noted (and discussed) of the patient's current versus past ability to self-calm. The therapist and patient together explore and decide what specific coping, self-calming strategies the patient will continue to use or experiment with between sessions.

In the next 60 minutes or so, the patient reexperiences the traumatic imagery (imaginal exposure), rescripts the traumatic imagery (develops mastery imagery), and develops ADULT–CHILD imagery. Each phase of imagery follows the same format and begins with the same traumatic memory as in session 1, as the therapist's approach remains primarily facilitative and nondirective.

After the patient has completed the exposure, mastery, and ADULT–CHILD imagery phases, and has had several moments to adapt to the completion of the imagery, the therapist administers the PIQ-A, facilitates processing and debriefing of the imagery session, and reviews the safety contract (if applicable).

Discuss Writing a Follow-Up Letter

The therapist introduces the idea of writing a follow-up letter either to the perpetrator or to another individual (e.g., mother) who the survivor feels was an intricate part of the traumatic experience. The patient is again asked to express current thoughts and feelings about the experience to this individual. The rationale for writing a follow-up letter may be explained as follows:

> Trauma survivors' thoughts and feelings about their experience tend to evolve or even change during treatment. Writing a follow-up letter to the perpetrator, or to another individual who may have been a silent partner or accomplice, offers survivors an opportunity to catch up with their current emotional processing of the trauma, as well as to work through and verbally process any remaining thoughts and feelings. How would you feel about writing a follow-up letter this week as part of your homework?

The therapist allows sufficient time to discuss and process reactions to the proposed assignment and makes sure the patient understands that the letter is *not* to be sent.

Homework Assignment (Session 4)

I. Process further your reactions to today's imagery session.
   1. Listen daily to the audiotape of the entire imagery ses-

sion (exposure and rescripting).
   2. Record your SUDs on the Homework Record both prior to and after listening to the audiotaped imagery session.
   3. Fill out the PIQ-A and record the PIQ score on the Homework Record immediately after listening to the audiotaped imagery session.
   4. Write out your personal reactions to the audiotaped imagery session in a journal.
   5. Record on the Traumatic Flashback Incident Record any recurring flashbacks or nightmares experienced between sessions.

II. Document efforts to self-calm and self-soothe.

Each time you feel upset and attempt to self-calm, write down the following information:
   1. the upsetting situation;
   2. the level of distress felt (on a 1 to 10 scale) immediately before and after efforts to self-calm;
   3. the upsetting thoughts and images;
   4. the specific interventions that you attempted (such as self-calming imagery, calling a friend, working out);
   5. how successful each intervention was.

III. Write a follow-up letter.

Write a follow-up letter to the perpetrator or to another individual toward whom you have strong emotional reactions about your traumatic experiences. Do not send the letter, but bring it to the next session for processing.

IV. Bring homework to next session for review.

SESSION 5

Assess general mood and between-session mood shifts
Review homework
    Discuss follow-up letter to perpetrator
    Review reactions to daily audiotape listening

Review efficacy of self-calming strategies attempted
Facilitate imaginal exposure, mastery imagery, and ADULT–CHILD imagery
Administer Post-Imagery Questionnaire-A (PIQ-A)
Process and debrief
Review contract for safety (if applicable)
Assign homework

Allow two hours for session 5. The first few minutes are spent reviewing the patient's general mood, between-session shifts in mood, reactions to the previous session, and homework. The patient is encouraged to read aloud and discuss the letter addressed to the perpetrator. (Again it may be useful to discuss with the patient at this point the possibility of incorporating information from the letter into the imagery later in the session.) Once the letter to the perpetrator has been adequately processed, the therapist and patient then review in detail the remainder of the homework together, beginning with the Homework Record and the Traumatic Flashback Incident Record. Again the patient's SUDs data and PIQ scores—as well as the presence, frequency, and intensity of flashbacks—are compared with data from previous sessions. Progress, or lack of progress, in these areas is noted and specific problems are identified and discussed with the patient if necessary.

The therapist again inquires about the patient's ability between sessions to self-calm and self-soothe when feeling upset, and reviews the efficacy of the self-calming strategies that the patient has attempted. The therapist and patient together explore and decide what specific coping, self-calming strategies the patient will continue to use or experiment with between sessions.

In the next 60 minutes or so, the patient reexperiences the traumatic imagery (imaginal exposure), rescripts the traumatic imagery (develops mastery imagery), and develops ADULT–CHILD imagery. Each phase of imagery follows the same format and begins with the same traumatic memory as in session 1. The therapist's approach remains primarily facilitative and nondirective. Once the patient has completed the exposure, mastery, and ADULT–CHILD imagery phases, and has had several moments to adapt to the completion of the imagery, the therapist administers the PIQ-A, and facilitates processing and debriefing of the imagery session.

Homework Assignment (Session 5)

I. Process further your reactions to today's imagery session.
   1. Listen daily to the audiotape of the entire imagery session (exposure and rescripting).
   2. Record your SUDs on the Homework Record both prior to and after listening to the audiotaped imagery session.
   3. Fill out the PIQ-A and record the PIQ score on the Homework Record immediately after listening to the audiotaped imagery session.
   4. Write out your personal reactions to the audiotaped imagery session in a journal.
   5. Record on the Traumatic Flashback Incident Record any recurring flashbacks or nightmares experienced between sessions.

II. Document efforts to self-calm and self-soothe.

Each time you feel upset and attempt to self-calm, write down the following information:
   1. the upsetting situation;
   2. the level of distress felt (on a 1 to 10 scale) immediately before and after efforts to self-calm;
   3. the upsetting thoughts and images;
   4. the specific interventions that you attempted (such as self-calming imagery, calling a friend, going on a long walk, working out);
   5. how successful each intervention was.

III. Bring homework to next session for review.

SESSION 6

Assess general mood and between-session mood shifts
Review homework
> Review Homework Record and Traumatic Flashback Incident Record data
> Review efficacy of self-calming strategies
> Explore application of additional self-calming/coping strategies to current life stressors and upsetting situations

Review safety contract (if applicable)
Assign Homework

Allow 90 minutes for session 6. The first few minutes are spent reviewing the patient's general mood, between-session shifts in moods, and reactions to the previous session. The therapist and patient then review in detail the homework together, beginning with the Homework Record and the Traumatic Flashback Incident Record. The SUDs data and PIQ scores—as well as the presence, frequency, and intensity of flashbacks/nightmares—are compared with data from previous sessions. Progress, or lack of progress, in these areas is noted and specific problems are identified and discussed if necessary.

The therapist inquires about the patient's ability between sessions to self-calm and self-soothe, especially when feeling upset, and reviews the efficacy of the self-calming strategies attempted. The therapist and patient together explore and identify current stressors or upsetting situations in the patient's life and decide what specific coping, self-calming strategies the patient might use or experiment with between sessions.

Homework Assignment (Session 6)

 I. Record on the Traumatic Flashback Incident Record flashbacks or nightmares experienced between sessions.

 II. Document efforts to self-calm and self-soothe.

Each time you feel upset and attempt to self-calm, write down the following information:

1. the upsetting situation;
2. the level of distress felt (on a 1 to 10 scale) immediately before and after efforts to self-calm;
3. the upsetting thoughts and images;
4. the specific interventions that you attempted (such as self-calming imagery, calling a friend, going on a long walk, working out);
5. the effectiveness of each intervention attempted:

    a. rate the effectiveness of each intervention using a 0 to 100 scale

    >0 = not at all successful
    100 = completely successful

    b. explore how the effectiveness of each intervention might be improved.

III. Bring homework to next session for review.

SESSION 7

Assess general mood and between-session mood shifts
Review homework
>Review Traumatic Flashback Incident Record data
Review efficacy of coping, self-calming strategies
Explore application of additional self-calming/coping strategies to current life stressors and upsetting situations.
Conduct mid-treatment review
Review safety contract (if applicable)
Assign homework

Allow 90 minutes for session 7. The first few minutes are spent reviewing the patient's general mood, between-session shifts in moods, and reactions to the previous session. The therapist and patient then review the homework together, beginning with the Traumatic Flashback Incident Record. The presence, frequency, and intensity of flashbacks/nightmares are compared with data from previous sessions. The therapist and patient review the efficacy of self-calming strategies attempted since last session and collaboratively determine what specific coping, self-calming strategies the patient will continue to use or experiment with.

The therapist also explains that an important focus of the homework in the next phase of treatment will include identifying, and coping more effectively with, current stressors and stressful situations in the patient's life, and that the out-of-session efforts to self-calm will be integrated as part of stress-reducing, coping strategies. The therapist and patient then collaboratively identify a specific, distressing situation (which the patient is currently facing) and explore possible coping, self-calming strategies that the patient may implement between sessions (e.g., journaling, engaging in relaxation imagery or focused breathing, calling a friend, using a computer, going for a walk, working out). It is important, however, that the coping/self-calming strategies initially come from the patient and not from the therapist, because what the clinician may consider to be a self-calming strategy (e.g., relaxation training, focused breathing) may in fact trigger emotional distress (e.g., traumatic flashbacks) in some patients. This may be facilitated by asking the patient what strategies she has successfully used in the past when attempting to cope with stressful situations.

Before homework is assigned, a brief mid-treatment review is conducted in which the patient's reactions (general and specific) to treatment thus far are invited, discussed, and processed. The therapist takes this opportunity to again reinforce the work that the patient is doing, offer reassurance, and point out specific areas of progress. If necessary, the safety contract is reviewed and the patient is reminded to call the therapist between sessions if strong urges to self-abuse or self-harm arise.

Homework Assignment (Session 7)

I. Record on the Traumatic Flashback Incident Record flashbacks or nightmares experienced between sessions.

II. Document efforts to cope with stressful/upsetting situations.

When you find yourself in an upsetting/stressful situation, write down the following:

1. the upsetting situation and specific stressor;
2. the level of distress you feel (on a 1 to 10 scale) immediately before and after efforts to self-calm;
3. the specific upsetting thoughts and images you have while in the stressful situation;
4. how you attempt to self-calm while in the upsetting situation;
5. how you attempt to cope with the situation;
6. how successful your efforts are to self-calm and cope with the upsetting situation;
7. additional coping strategies you might consider using the next time you are faced with a similar stressful situation.

III. Bring homework to next session for review.

SESSION 8

Assess general mood and between-session mood shifts
Review homework
    Review Traumatic Flashback Incident Record
    Review efforts to self-calm and effectively cope with stressful/upsetting situations
Facilitate imaginal exposure, mastery imagery, and ADULT–CHILD imagery follow-up
Administer Post-Imagery Questionnaire-A
Process and debrief
Determine if additional exposure and rescripting sessions of the traumatic imagery are indicated

Introduce additional guidelines for crisis management
Review safety contract (if applicable)
Assign homework

Allow two hours for session 8. The first few minutes are spent reviewing the patient's general mood, between-session shifts in moods, and reactions to the previous session. The therapist and patient then review the homework together, beginning with the Traumatic Flashback Incident Record. The presence, frequency, and intensity of flashbacks and nightmares since the last session are compared with data from previous sessions.

The therapist also inquires about the patient's ability between sessions to cope with stressful situations and to self-calm when feeling upset, and reviews the efficacy of these strategies. The therapist and patient collaboratively explore and decide what specific self-calming, stress-reducing coping strategies the patient will continue to use or experiment with.

Exposure, Mastery, and Adult-Child Imagery Follow-Up

The therapist then explains the need for doing a follow-up imagery session of the traumatic event to determine the patient's readiness to proceed to the next imagery phase of treatment. The therapist thus facilitates the patient's reexperiencing the traumatic imagery (imaginal exposure), rescripting the traumatic imagery (mastery imagery), and developing ADULT–CHILD imagery. Each phase of imagery follows the same format and the same traumatic memory as in sessions 1 to 5, as the therapist's approach remains facilitative and nondirective. After the patient has completed the exposure, mastery, and ADULT–CHILD imagery phases, and has had several moments to adapt to the completion of the imagery, the therapist administers the PIQ-A and facilitates processing and debriefing of the imagery session.

Criteria for Progressing to the ADULT–CHILD Only Imagery Phase

After the above imagery session has been completed and adequately processed, the patient's readiness to proceed to the imagery phase is assessed. Generally, the following criteria should be met before the patient is deemed ready for the nonexposure/ADULT–CHILD only imagery phase:

1. The patient has adequately processed, and become relatively desensitized to, the traumatic imagery.
2. During master imagery, the patient's ADULT no longer experiences difficulty confronting the perpetrator and rescuing the CHILD, and is no longer terrified of the perpetrator while rescuing the CHILD.

If, in the follow-up imagery session, the patient's ADULT continues to experience difficulty confronting the perpetrator and rescuing the CHILD, or is still very afraid of the perpetrator while rescuing the CHILD (i.e., has a score of 50 or greater on item 3 or 4 of the Post-Imagery Questionnaire-A), then subsequent sessions should continue with the session 5 imagery format, which includes exposure to, and rescripting of, the traumatic imagery, until the ADULT feels sufficiently empowered vis-à-vis the perpetrator.

When the therapist and patient agree that the patient is indeed ready to move on to the nonexposure phase of treatment, the therapist reiterates that the focus of the remaining imagery sessions, beginning next session, will be on ADULT–CHILD only imagery. Should difficulties arise during the ADULT–CHILD only imagery (e.g., the perpetrator enters the ADULT–CHILD imagery scene), the clinician may wish to include some additional abuse imagery (exposure and rescripting) sessions. As previously mentioned, it is crucial that the therapist refer to this phase as ADULT–CHILD imagery, not as adult–nurturing–child imagery. This is especially important when the ADULT is still harboring hostile thoughts and feelings toward the CHILD, such as anger, blame, or hate, that may need to be expressed directly to the CHILD before any genuine nurturing toward the CHILD can be felt and expressed.

Guidelines for Crisis Management

The safety contract is reviewed and reinforced, and the patient is reminded to call the therapist if a crisis arises or serious difficulties are encountered. Before placing a crisis call to the therapist, however, the patient is instructed henceforth to first visualize and write out (preferably in a journal) an imaginary conversation with the therapist, in which the patient

1. describes the upsetting situation,
2. verbalizes active thoughts and feelings about the situation,
3. describes to the therapist (in imagery) how she has already attempted to cope with the situation,
4. "listens" carefully to the therapist's response and attentively writes down what she "hears" the therapist saying.

If, after having this imaginary conversation with the therapist, the patient still feels the need to call, she may do so. However, the patient is informed that upon making such a call, the therapist's initial response will be to ask for a report on (1) whether the patient carried out an imaginary conversation with the therapist, (2) what the patient has written down from that imaginary conversation, and (3) what the patient "saw" and "heard" in the therapist's response.

Development of Positive Therapist Introjects

Because victims of childhood trauma and abuse tend to have such hostile and self-abusive introjects (akin to negative self-schemas), the cognitive-behavioral guidelines for crisis management described above can be useful in helping patients develop a positive therapist introject that competes with, and eventually replaces, their heretofore negative introjects. (Henry and colleagues [1990] discuss the formation of introjects and the relationship between the development of positive therapist introjects and good psychotherapy outcome.) The new therapist introject is essentially a positive internal representation of the therapist that, when activated or summoned up by the patient, can have a calming/soothing effect on the patient's mood, especially during times of emotional distress, and that eventually becomes a permanent part of the patient's schematic internal representation of self.

Homework Assignment (Session 8)

I. Process further your reactions to today's imagery session.
   1. Listen daily to the audiotape of the entire imagery session.
   2. Record your SUDs on the Homework Record both prior to and after listening to the audiotaped imagery session.
   3. Fill out the PIQ-A and record the PIQ score on the Homework Record immediately after listening to the audiotaped imagery session.
   4. Write out your personal reactions to the audiotaped imagery session in a journal.

II. Record on the Traumatic Flashback Incident Record flashbacks or nightmares experienced between sessions.

III. Document efforts to cope with stressful/upsetting situations.

When in upsetting/stressful situations, write out the following:

1. the upsetting situation and specific stressor;
2. the level of distress felt (on a 1 to 10 scale);
3. the specific upsetting thoughts, feelings, and images you have while in the stressful situation;
4. how you attempt to self-calm while in the upsetting situation;
5. how you attempt to cope with the situation;
6. how successful your efforts are to self-calm and cope with the upsetting situation;
7. other strategies you might consider when attempting to cope with such stressful situations in the future.

V. Bring homework to next session for review.

5

Self-Nurturing Imagery Only

SESSION 9

Assess general mood and between-session mood shifts
Conduct brief mid-treatment review
    Review homework
    Review reactions to daily audiotape listening
    Review Traumatic Flashback Incident Record data
    Review efforts to self-calm and cope with stressful/upsetting situations
Confirm readiness to progress to nonexposure imagery phase
Develop adult-nurturing-child imagery
Administer Post-Imagery Questionnaire-B (PIQ-B)
Process and debrief
Review safety contract (if applicable)
Assign homework

Allow 90 minutes for session 9. The first few minutes are spent reviewing the patient's general mood, between-session shifts in moods, and reactions to the previous session. A brief mid-treatment review is then conducted in which the patient's reactions (general and specific) to treatment thus far are invited, discussed, and processed. The therapist takes this opportunity to reinforce the difficult but beneficial work that the patient is doing, point out specific areas of progress and growth, and offer encouragement and reassurance.

After discussing general reactions to the homework, the therapist and patient review the homework in detail, beginning with the patient's reactions to the audiotape of the previous imagery session, including the Homework Record, the SUDs data and PIQ scores, and the patient's written journal. The therapist inquires about the presence, frequency, and intensity of flashbacks and nightmares since last session, and reviews the data recorded on the Traumatic Flashback Incident Record. The SUDs data, PIQ scores, and flashback data are compared with data from previous sessions. Progress is noted and specific problems are identified and discussed if necessary.

The therapist inquires about the patient's ability since last session to cope with stressful situations and to self-calm when feeling upset, and reviews the efficacy of these strategies. The therapist and patient collaboratively explore and decide what specific self-calming, stress-reducing coping strategies the patient will continue to use or experiment with.

Once the homework has been adequately reviewed and processed, the therapist confirms the patient's readiness to progress to the nonexposure imagery phase. The patient is reminded that the focus of the remaining imagery sessions will be on ADULT–CHILD imagery only, and that the traumatic imagery will no longer be reexperienced or rescripted.

Adult-Nurturing-Child Imagery

During the next hour or so, the therapist facilitates the development of adult-nurturing-child imagery. The therapist refers to this phase as "ADULT–CHILD imagery." Instead of beginning with exposure to the traumatic imagery, as was done in sessions 1 to 5, the imagery session now begins with the patient visually "checking in" with the CHILD. The therapist begins this phase as follows:

> When you are ready, you may close your eyes and visually "check in" with the CHILD.

The therapist facilitates the adult-nurturing-child imagery by asking:

> Where is the CHILD?
> What is the CHILD doing?
> How is the CHILD feeling?
> Where are you, the ADULT, in relation to the CHILD?
> How far are you, the ADULT, from the CHILD?
> Does the CHILD see you, the ADULT?
> How does the CHILD respond to your presence?
> How do you, the ADULT, respond to the CHILD's presence?
> How are you, the ADULT, feeling?
> What would you, the ADULT, like to do or say to the CHILD?
> Can you do/say that to the CHILD directly?
> How does the CHILD respond?
> When you look directly into the CHILD's eyes, what do you see?
> How do you react to what you see in the CHILD's eyes?

At this point in treatment, many patients visualize themselves as an ADULT holding, hugging, and offering nurturance to the CHILD. If positive images of the CHILD and ADULT interacting emerge, this is generally viewed as a good prognostic indicator, and the therapist facilitates, through Socratic imagery, the further development of such images. If, however, the ADULT has continued difficulty nurturing the CHILD, feels ambivalent toward the CHILD, blames the CHILD, or wants to hurt or abandon the CHILD, it is important that the ADULT express such negative feelings directly to the CHILD from close proximity. Again, with more severely disturbed patients, such intimate ADULT–CHILD exchanges may activate an unlovable schema, which in turn can provide a unique therapeutic opportunity to visually and verbally confront this highly treatment-resistant schema within the context of a supportive, therapeutic context. In many instances, as the ADULT moves closer to the CHILD in physical proximity, the ADULT becomes more "taken in" by the CHILD's pain, which evokes strong feelings toward the CHILD that are empathic, apologetic, or conciliatory in nature. (See Chapter 4 for specific questions the therapist may ask to facilitate such ADULT–CHILD interactions.)

Once it appears that the ADULT has offered sufficient nurturance to the CHILD and the patient may be ready to end the imagery, the therapist asks:

> Is there anything more that you, the ADULT, would like to do or say to the CHILD before bringing the imagery to a close?

When the patient indicates a readiness to terminate the imagery session, the therapist responds:

> You may now let the imagery fade away, and when you are ready, you may open your eyes.

Administering the Post-Imagery Questionnaire-B

After the patient has had several moments to adapt to the completion of the imagery phase, the therapist administers the Post-Imagery Questionnaire-B (PIQ-B) (Appendix B), which involves reading each item aloud to the patient and recording the patient's numerical rating on the line to the left of each item. The PIQ-B is used to obtain immediate patient feedback about the imagery session just experienced as well as to monitor session-by-session progress for the remaining imagery sessions.

Processing and Debriefing

After the PIQ-B has been administered, reactions to the imagery session are discussed and processed together with the patient. To facilitate such processing, the therapist may ask:

> How was that for you?
> How are you feeling now?
> What did you see when you looked into the CHILD's eyes?
> What were you thinking and feeling when you looked into the CHILD's eyes?
> How are you feeling now toward the CHILD?

As reactions to the imagery session are invited, discussed, and processed, the therapist continues to look for opportunities to reinforce the work the patient is doing, offer reassurance, and point out specific areas of progress both within and outside of the imagery sessions. The safety contract is reviewed and reinforced, and the patient is reminded to call the therapist between sessions if strong urges to self-abuse or self-harm arise.

Homework Assignment (Session 9)
   I. Process further your reactions to today's imagery session.
      1. Listen daily to the audiotape of the imagery session.
      2. Record your SUDs on the Homework Record both prior to and after listening to the audiotaped imagery session.

3. Fill out the PIQ-B and record the PIQ score on the Homework Record immediately after listening to the audiotaped imagery session.

II. Record on the Traumatic Flashback Incident Record flashbacks and nightmares experienced between sessions.

III. Document efforts to cope with stressful/upsetting situations.

When in an upsetting/stressful situation, write down the following:

1. the upsetting situation and specific stressor;
2. the level of distress felt (on a 1 to 10 scale);
3. the specific upsetting thoughts, feelings, and images you have while in the stressful situation;
4. how you attempt to self-calm while in the upsetting situation;
5. how you attempt to cope with the situation;
6. how successful your efforts are to self-calm and cope with the upsetting situation;
7. other strategies you might consider when attempting to cope with such stressful situations in the future.

IV. Bring homework to next session for review.

SESSIONS 10 TO 12

Assess general mood and between-session mood shifts
Review homework
    Review reactions to daily audiotape listening
    Review Traumatic Flashback Incident Record data
    Review efforts to self-calm and cope with stressful/upsetting situations
Develop adult-nurturing-child imagery
Administer Post-Imagery Questionnaire-B (PIQ-B)
Process and debrief
Review safety contract (if applicable)
Assign homework

Allow 90 minutes for each session. The first few minutes are spent reviewing the patient's general mood, between-session shifts in moods, reactions to the previous session, and general reactions to the homework. The therapist and patient then review each homework assignment, beginning with the patient's daily reactions to the audiotape of the previous imagery session, including the Homework Record, the SUDs data and PIQ scores, and the patient's written journal. The therapist inquires about the presence, frequency, and intensity of flashbacks and nightmares since the previous session and reviews the data recorded on the Traumatic Flashback Incident Record. The SUDs data, PIQ scores, and flashback data are compared with data from previous sessions. Progress is noted and specific problems are identified and discussed if necessary.

The therapist inquires about the patient's ability since the previous session to cope with stressful situations and to self-calm when feeling upset, and reviews the efficacy of these efforts. The therapist and patient collaboratively explore and decide what specific self-calming, stress-reducing coping strategies the patient will continue to use or experiment with between sessions.

Adult-Nurturing-Child Imagery

During the next hour or so, the therapist again facilitates the development of adult-nurturing-child imagery (as specified in session 8). Once it appears that the ADULT has offered sufficient nurturance to the CHILD and the patient may be ready to end the imagery, the therapist asks:

> Is there anything more that you, the ADULT, would like to do or say to the CHILD before bringing the imagery to a close?

When the patient has indicated a readiness to terminate the imagery session, the therapist responds:

You may now let the imagery fade away, and when you are ready, you may open your eyes.

Administering the Post-Imagery Questionnaire-B

After the patient has had several moments to adapt to the completion of the imagery phase, the therapist administers the Post-Imagery Questionnaire-B (PIQ-B). The PIQ-B data are used to obtain immediate patient feedback about the imagery session just experienced and to monitor session-by-session progress.

Processing and Debriefing

After the PIQ-B has been administered, reactions to the imagery session are discussed and processed with the patient. The therapist continues to portray a positive and reassuring demeanor vis-à-vis the patient, while reinforcing specific areas of progress as well as articulating areas with which the patient is still struggling. If applicable, the safety contract continues to be reviewed and reinforced, and the patient is reminded to call the therapist between sessions if strong urges to self-abuse or self-harm arise.

Homework Assignment (Sessions 10–12)

I. Process further your reactions to today's imagery session.
   1. Listen daily to the audiotape of the imagery session.
   2. Record your SUDs on the Homework Record both prior to and after listening to the audiotaped imagery session.
   3. Fill out the PIQ-B and record the PIQ score on the Homework Record immediately after listening to the audiotaped imagery session.
   4. Write out your personal reactions to the audiotaped imagery session in a journal.

II. Record on the Traumatic Flashback Incident Record flashbacks and nightmares experienced between sessions.

III. Document efforts to cope with stressful/upsetting situations.

When you find yourself in an upsetting/stressful situation, write down the following:

1. the upsetting situation and specific stressor;
2. the specific upsetting thoughts and images you have while in the stressful situation;
3. the level of distress felt (on a 1 to 10 scale) immediately before and after efforts to self-calm;
4. how you attempt to self-calm while in the upsetting situation;
5. how you attempt to cope with the situation;
6. how successful your efforts are to self-calm and cope with the upsetting situation;
7. other possible ways you might attempt to cope (think, feel, and act) while in such a stressful situation.

IV. Bring homework to next session for review.

SESSION 13

Assess general mood and between-session mood shifts
Review homework
    Review reactions to daily audiotape listening
    Review Traumatic Flashback Incident Record data
    Review efficacy of self-calming/stress-reducing coping strategies
Develop adult-nurturing-child imagery
Administer Post-Imagery Questionnaire-B
Process and debrief
Introduce next phase of treatment: a higher order cognitive/linguistic processing
Review safety contract (if applicable)
Assign homework

Allow two hours for session 13. The first few minutes are spent reviewing the patient's general mood, between-session shifts in moods, reactions to the previous session, and general reactions to the homework. The therapist and patient then review each homework assignment together, beginning with the patient's daily reactions to the audiotape of the last imagery session, including the Homework Record, the daily SUDs data and PIQ scores, and the patient's written journal. The therapist inquires about the presence, frequency, and intensity of flashbacks and nightmares since the previous session and reviews the data recorded on the Traumatic Flashback Incident Record. The SUDs data, PIQ scores, and flashback/nightmare data are compared with data from previous sessions. The therapist and patient then review progress made during the adult-nurturing-child phase of imagery.

The therapist inquires about the patient's ability since last session to cope with stressful situations and to self-calm when feeling upset, and reviews the efficacy of these efforts. The patient is encouraged to continue with self-calming imagery and daily journaling. Specific current stressors in the patient's life are identified, stress-reducing coping strategies are discussed and rehearsed (if applicable), and plans for how to handle possible future crisis situations are discussed.

Adult-Nurturing-Child Imagery

The therapist facilitates the development of adult-nurturing-child imagery over the next 30 to 60 minutes. Once it appears that the ADULT has offered sufficient nurturance to the CHILD and the patient may be ready to end the imagery, the therapist asks:

> Is there anything more that you, the ADULT, would like to do or say to the CHILD before bringing the imagery to a close?

SELF-NURTURING IMAGERY ONLY

When the patient indicates a readiness to terminate the imagery session, the therapist responds:

You may now let the imagery fade away, and when you are ready, you may open your eyes.

After the patient has had several moments to adapt to the completion of the imagery session, the therapist administers the PIQ-B. The therapist uses the PIQ-B to obtain immediate patient feedback about the imagery session just experienced and to ascertain overall progress. As reactions to the imagery session are discussed and processed, the patient is reminded that today's imagery session is the last scheduled ADULT–CHILD imagery session at this time. The therapist and patient then review progress to date, as well as progress made during this ADULT–CHILD only phase of imagery.

Homework Assignment (Session 13)

I. Process further your reactions to today's imagery session.
   1. Listen daily to the audiotape of the imagery session.
   2. Record your SUDs on the Homework Record both prior to and after listening to the audiotaped imagery session.
   3. Fill out the PIQ-B and record the PIQ score on the Homework Record immediately after listening to the audiotaped imagery session.
   4. Write out your personal reactions to the audiotaped imagery session in a journal.

II. Record on the Traumatic Flashback Incident Record flashbacks and nightmares experienced between sessions.

III. Document efforts to cope with stressful/upsetting situations.

   When you find yourself in an upsetting/stressful situation, write down the following:

1. the upsetting situation and specific stressor;
2. the specific upsetting thoughts and feelings you have while in the stressful situation;
3. the level of distress felt (on a 1 to 10 scale) immediately before and after efforts to self-calm;
4. how you attempt to self-calm while in the upsetting situation;
5. how you attempt to cope with the situation;
6. how effective your efforts are to self-calm and cope with the upsetting situation;
7. other strategies you might consider when attempting to cope with such stressful situations in the future.

IV. Bring all homework to next session for review and processing.

6
A Higher Order Cognitive/Linguistic Processing

SESSION 14

Assess general mood and between-session mood shifts
Review homework
    Review reactions to daily audiotape listening
    Review Traumatic Flashback Incident Record data
    Review efficacy of self-calming/stress-reducing coping strategies
Begin next phase of treatment: a higher order cognitive/linguistic processing
Review safety contract (if applicable)
Assign homework

Allow 90 minutes for session 14. The first few minutes are spent reviewing the patient's general mood, between-session shifts in moods, reactions to the previous session, and general reactions to the homework. The therapist and patient then review each homework assignment together, beginning with patient's daily reactions to the audiotape of the last imagery session, including the Homework Record, the daily SUDs data and PIQ scores, and the patient's written journal. The therapist inquires about the presence, frequency, and intensity of flashbacks and nightmares since the previous session and reviews the data recorded on the Traumatic Flashback Incident Record. The SUDs data, PIQ scores, and flashback/nightmare data are compared with data from previous sessions. The therapist and patient then review progress made during the adult-nurturing-child phase of imagery and discuss whether additional ADULT–CHILD imagery sessions might be beneficial at a later time.

The therapist inquires about the patient's ability since last session to cope with stressful situations and to self-calm when feeling upset, and reviews the efficacy of these efforts. The patient is encouraged to continue with self-calming imagery and daily journaling. Specific current stressors in the patient's life are identified, stress-reducing coping strategies are discussed and rehearsed (if applicable), and plans for how to handle possible future crisis situations are discussed.

Beginning the Next Phase of Treatment

The therapist reiterates that the next phase of treatment focuses on a higher order processing of the patient's traumas, the goal of which is to get beyond the victimization by both accepting it as part of the patient's life experiences and transforming it into a meaningful cognitive frame. The patient is informed that a vital part of this higher order processing involves a number of writing and reading assignments. The therapist then facilitates a discussion about how the victimization experiences have shaped the patient's entire belief system and worldview, including attribution of life events and core beliefs (schemas) about self, others, and relationships, and whether the patient might be willing to reexamine these traumagenic core beliefs. This discussion should be kept relatively brief as the patient is encouraged to continue processing such victimization-related questions as part of the homework. The safety contract is again reviewed, if applicable.

Homework Assignment (Session 14)

I. What does your victimization mean to you, past and present?

1. Write about your victimization—how you were unfairly treated, exploited, abused, abandoned, and traumatized.
2. How has your victimization affected your beliefs about yourself, your beliefs about others, your beliefs about relationships, and your beliefs about life?
3. How has your victimization influenced your views on
   a. safety
   b. trust
   c. worth
   d. power
   e. competence
   f. intimacy

   (adapted from McCann and Pearlman 1990).

4. As a child, whom did you blame for your victimization? Please explain.
   a. How much did you blame the perpetrator(s)? Why?
   b. How much did you blame yourself? Why?
   c. Were there others whom you blamed for your victimization? Who were they? Why were they to blame?

5. As an adult today, whom do you blame for your victimization? Please explain.
   a. How much do you blame the perpetrator(s) today for your victimization? Why?
   b. How much do you blame yourself today for your victimization? Why?
   c. Are there others whom you blame today for your victimization? Who are they? Why are they to blame?

6. How much anger do you feel today about your childhood victimization? Please elaborate.

a. How much anger do you feel toward the perpetrator(s)?
b. How much anger do you feel toward yourself?
c. How much anger do you feel toward others?
d. What do you do with the anger you feel toward the perpetrator? Toward yourself? Toward others?
e. Are there constructive ways you have found to channel your anger?

7. How has your victimization affected your religious/spiritual views?

II. What do you know about your perpetrator(s)?

1. What thoughts and feelings do you have about the nature and character of your perpetrator(s)?
2. What do you know about the family background of your perpetrator(s)?
3. What could possess a person to commit such cruel and vicious acts against another human being?

III. Please address the following questions relating to the thoughts, feelings, and behaviors you experience when you are in "victim space" versus "survivor space" and whether these are open to modification.

1. Are you destined to think, feel, and act like a victim for the rest of your life? Please elaborate.
2. How much of the time are you in victim space (i.e., feel like a victim) versus in survivor space?
3. When you are in victim space, how do you think, feel, and act?
4. When you are in survivor space (i.e., *not* in victim space), how do you think, feel, and act?
5. What are the pros and cons of being in victim space?
6. What are the pros and cons of being in survivor space?
7. What would need to happen or change in order for you to stop thinking of yourself as a victim?
8. If you viewed yourself as someone other than a victim, how would you view yourself?

IV. Bring homework to next session for review.

SESSION 15

Assess general mood and between-session mood shifts
Review reactions to previous session
Review homework
    Review Traumatic Flashback Incident Record data
    Review and process the written responses to each item of the victimization/survivor homework
    Look for opportunities to confront traumatogenic schemas
Introduce Frankl's *Man's Search for Meaning*
Review safety contract (if applicable)
Assign homework

Allow 90 minutes for session 15. The first few minutes are spent reviewing the patient's general mood, between-session mood shifts, reactions to the previous session, and general reactions to the homework. The therapist briefly inquires about the presence, frequency, and intensity of flashbacks and nightmares since last session, and reviews the data recorded on the Traumatic Flashback Incident Record.

The therapist and patient then together carefully review and process the patient's written responses to each item of the victimization/survivor homework. The patient's responses to these items may reveal a great deal about the progress that the patient has made vis-à-vis specific trauma-related beliefs, attributions, and core schemas (e.g., powerlessness, unlovability, victimization, self-hatred/self-blame), as well as offer the clinician a clearer idea of the focus and duration of continued treatment. As the victimization-related written responses are reviewed and processed, the therapist uses a primarily Socratic questioning approach to challenge the patient's maladaptive beliefs. The following are examples of the kind of questions the therapist may ask in this context:

Help me understand how a young child could be blamed for the abuse that was perpetrated on her.

Do you feel that other victims of childhood abuse are also to blame for the abuse they experienced?

How is it then that other victims of childhood abuse are not to blame, and you are?

Are you saying that you have a double standard? Help me understand the rationale behind that.

How is it that you are bad, unlovable, and worthless because of what a disturbed, sadistic individual did to you? Help me understand that.

It is important to spend sufficient time reviewing how the abuse experiences have affected the patient's views on safety, trust, worth, power, competence, and intimacy, and to search collaboratively with the patient for evidence (past and present) that contradicts the patient's maladaptive beliefs on these dimensions. Considerable time may also need to be spent on examining and challenging patient beliefs relating to (1) whom the patient today blames or holds responsible for the traumatic experiences, (2) the degree and intensity of anger the patient feels toward the perpetrator versus self for the traumatic events, (3) how the patient channels such anger and toward whom it is directed, and (4) how the patient's religious or spiritual views have been affected by the traumas. Reviewing carefully the patient's responses to the perpetrator's nature, family background, and possible motivation for committing such cruel and vicious acts against another can shed additional light on the patient's trauma-related attributions.

There is a wide range of emotional responses in addition to anger that adult survivors of childhood trauma commonly experience, such as sadness, depression, anxiety, fear, and grief. It is important to listen to, process, and normalize patients' emotional responses to their traumas. Above all, it is important to validate again and again patients' victimization experiences, while at the same time challenging victims to move beyond their victimization and not get stuck in "victim space." The therapist needs to be sensitive and supportive while urging patients to carefully weigh the pros and cons of being in victim space, and challenging them to imagine or describe how they might view and live their lives differently if they stopped viewing themselves as victims. Having patients verbalize, and put into writing, the specific thoughts and feelings that are activated when they are in victim space versus when they are in survivor space can be an enlightening exercise. Carefully weighing the costs and benefits of being in victim space versus being in survivor space can serve as a useful cognitive intervention in challenging victimization cognitions and underlying traumagenic schemas.

Identifying, Challenging, and Modifying Traumagenic Schemas

In confronting the patient's core traumagenic beliefs and schemas, the therapist's task is to aggressively challenge the validity of the patient's maladaptive beliefs and schemas while remaining supportive, sensitive, and understanding. In one instance, a therapist likened the patient's core schemas to little demons that brainwash the patient into thinking of herself as bad and evil and blaming herself for the abuse she suffered as a child:

> It's not you personally whom I am challenging or attacking. But I am going after, and attacking, those little demons inside your head who have convinced you that you are bad, evil, that the abuse was your fault, and that you are undeserving of anything good.

Schema modification can often be facilitated by identifying and activating the core beliefs and schemas as self-statements (e.g., "I am unlovable," "I deserved my abuse because I am such a bad, evil person," "I deserve to be punished," "I am a victim and will always be one," "I am unworthy of any happiness in my life"), giving them a label and a separate identity, and then challenging them via whatever means might be effective. Sometimes the therapist may need to be creative in finding effective means of confronting, challenging, and modifying the patient's maladaptive schemas.

While working with one adult survivor of severe childhood abuse (sexual and physical), the therapist confronted the patient's core traumagenic schemas by initially identifying her schema-emanating, negative self-talk as the "voices" in her head, and then activating the voices within the context of a humorous role play and making them sound silly, ridiculous, and not to be taken seriously. Specifically, the therapist role-played the patient's negative voices—which, the patient complained, had been flooding her thought processes daily—by repeating them aloud in a high-pitched, squeaky, chipmunk voice, to which the patient responded with near uncontrollable laughter. The following is a synopsis of their role play:

Therapist: (In squeaky, chipmunk voice) Okay, let me hear them voices. YOU HAVE NOTHING WORTHWHILE TO DO OR SAY. Let me hear you say it. Repeat after me. Go ahead, you have nothing to live for.

Client: (laughing) You have nothing worthwhile to say or do.

Therapist: That's right. You have nothing worthwhile to say or do. YOU NEED TO BE PUNISHED.

Client: You need to be punished (chuckling).

Therapist: You need to be punished, you're disgusting.

Client: You're disgusting.

Therapist: YOU'RE DISGUSTING! No one will come to your defense, you're not worth it.

Client: (laughing) No one will come to your defense, you're not worth it.

A HIGHER ORDER COGNITIVE/LINGUISTIC PROCESSING

Therapist: WHY ARE YOU LAUGHING? IT'S NOT FUNNY.

Client: You're so funny.

Therapist: But these are YOUR voices. You're disgusting, you have no right to exist.

Client: You're disgusting, you have no right to exist.

Therapist: YOU HAVE NO RIGHT TO EXIST. YOU'RE NOT GOOD ENOUGH TO BE WITH.

Client: You're not good enough to be with.

Therapist: Say it with a little more life. (In loud, even more exaggerated high-pitched, squeaky chipmunk voice) YOU'RE NOT GOOD ENOUGH TO BE WITH. YOU'RE DISGUSTING. NO ONE WANTS TO SPEND TIME WITH YOU. YOU NEED TO BE PUNISHED. Repeat after me. YOU NEED TO BE PUNISHED. Go ahead, give it your best shot!

Client: (laughing uncontrollably).

Therapist: YOU NEED TO BE PUNISHED.

Client: (still laughing) You need to be punished.

Therapist: You're disgusting... go ahead, try that one.

Client: (laughing so hard, she is barely able to talk) You're disgusting.

Therapist: (continues in high-pitched, squeaky voice) What's happening here? Look at me now. YOU HAVE NOTHING WORTHWHILE TO DO OR SAY. Repeat after me.

Client: (chuckling) You have nothing worthwhile to do or say.

Therapist: GOOD! YOU HAVE NO BLOODY RIGHT TO EXIST.

Client: (chuckling) You have no bloody right to exist.

An audiotape was made of the above role play, to which the patient listened daily for several weeks thereafter. The following is the patient's own account of the effect that this humorous role play had on the negative voices in her head:

Trying to control the voices [my negative self-talk], and not be controlled by them, has been an exhausting exercise in futility. Despite all the progress I had made in therapy, especially in mastering the abuse flashbacks, dealing with the voices felt hopeless, and it seemed like I would be stuck with them for the rest of my life. The image I get is that the voices become this sticky substance that gloms on to my brain cells and makes me feel tormented and so out of control. . . .

Listening to Dr. Smucker's tape this week where he takes on the character of the voices has created a light in darkness. Listening to the tape several times a day has changed the way I hear them [the voices]. Sometimes his change in voice sounded to me like the Wicked Witch of the West in *The Wizard of Oz* as she was being dissolved.

The sticky substance attacking my brain is starting to feel more fluid and movable. The voices in my head seem more manageable. His [Dr. Smucker's] voice now overrides the voices in my head. His voice makes me laugh, and the more I am able to laugh the less I feel the life being squeezed out of me. . . . There's comfort in his voice, even if it sounds goofy.

During stressful situations this past week I could hear Dr. Smucker's voice, even when I was not listening to the tape. Situations came up at work that were potentially explosive, but I consciously called up Dr. Smucker's voice and was able to move through the stressful situations without humiliating myself.

Searching for Meaning to Human Suffering

The therapist then invites a brief discussion on the topic of finding meaning in human suffering, by asking:

Can positive meaning be found in human suffering?
Is it possible for abuse and torture victims to become better people as a result of their suffering? Can you think of any examples?

How do these victims turn human-perpetrated tragedy and torture into a meaningful life experience?

The therapist may then suggest outside reading about victims of abuse and torture who have written about their experiences and their efforts to find meaning in their suffering. One such book that the therapist introduces is Viktor Frankl's *Man's Search for Meaning* (1959), in which Frankl writes about his experiences in the Nazi death camps during World War II and his search for meaning in the context of the unimaginable, human-perpetrated horrors to which he and others were subjected. The therapist then suggests that the patient read and process Frankl's book as part of the homework assignment for next time.

Homework Assignment (Session 15)

I. Read *Man's Search for Meaning* by Viktor Frankl.

  1. Write out your thoughts, feelings, and reactions to Frankl's account of his death camp experiences and his efforts to find meaning in them.
  2. Compare and contrast Frankl's death camp experiences to your own traumatic experiences. How are they similar? How are they different?

II. Record on the Traumatic Flashback Incident Record flashbacks and nightmares experienced between sessions.

III. Finish any uncompleted homework from last session.

IV. Bring homework to next session for review.

SESSION 16

Assess general mood and between-session mood shifts
Review reactions to previous session

Review homework
> Review Traumatic Flashback Incident Record data
> Review and process reactions to *Man's Search for Meaning* (an account of Frankl's death camp experiences)

Review safety contract (if applicable)
Assign homework

Allow 90 minutes for session 16. The first few minutes are spent reviewing the patient's general mood, between-session mood shifts, and reactions to the previous session. The therapist briefly inquires about the presence, frequency, and intensity of flashbacks and nightmares since last session, while reviewing the data recorded on the Traumatic Flashback Incident Record.

The remainder of the session is then focused on discussing and processing the patient's reactions to Frankl's book, *Man's Search for Meaning*. Specifically, the patient is asked to articulate how Frankl was able to survive and find meaning in the suffering he experienced and witnessed in the Nazi death camps (i.e., put these horrific events into a meaningful cognitive frame). The therapist may facilitate this by asking:

> How was Frankl able to maintain his integrity and emotionally survive the Nazi death camp?
>
> How was Frankl able to transform his experience of suffering in the death camp into an experience of meaning?
>
> How did Frankl's thoughts, feelings, and actions in the Nazi death camp compare and contrast with those of other concentration camp victims?

Search for Meaning to the Patient's Suffering

The therapist introduces the idea of searching for positive meaning to the patient's own suffering and may begin by sharing with the patient the following quote from Frankl:

> We must never forget that we may also find meaning in life even when confronted with a hopeless situation, when facing a fate that cannot be changed. For what then matters is to bear witness to the uniquely human potential at its best, which is to transform a personal tragedy into a triumph, to turn one's predicament into a human achievement. When we are no longer able to change a situation—just think of an incurable disease such as inoperable cancer—we are challenged to change ourselves. [p. 116]

The therapist may suggest the patient think about the traumatic experiences from two opposing viewpoints: (1) a Frankl viewpoint (i.e., How might Frankl frame your suffering had he had your experiences?), and (2) a non-Frankl viewpoint (i.e., How might someone stuck in victim mode frame your suffering?). The challenge for the therapist during such a discussion is to remain supportive of the patient while confronting the patient's maladaptive schemas/introjects.

While encouraging patients to find meaning in their suffering, the therapist may also emphasize that the search for meaning to one's existence is a lifelong human endeavor. As part of the homework, the patient is given a typewritten copy of the above Frankl quotation with instructions to put it in a highly visible place and to read it (and reflect on it) daily.

Homework Assignment (Session 16)

I. Read, and reflect on, the following quotation from Frankl every day before beginning with the written homework:

> We must never forget that we may also find meaning in life even when confronted with a hopeless situation, when facing a fate that cannot be changed. For what then matters is to bear witness to the uniquely human potential at its best, which is to transform a personal tragedy into a triumph, to turn one's predicament into a human achievement.

II. Search for positive meaning to your suffering.

  1. How would you view yourself, your life, and your suffering if

     a. you continued to think of yourself as a victim and remained stuck in your victimization?
     b. you were able to transform your suffering into meaningful life experiences?

III. Apply Frankl's perspective to your own life.

  1. If you applied Frankl's perspective to your own suffering, how would you view your experiences and your life differently? Please be specific.
  2. How might you be a better person today because of the suffering you experienced?
  3. How might you be able to contribute positively to the lives of others because of your suffering?
  4. Carry out the following experiment: on alternate days, give yourself permission to apply and live out Frankl's perspective to your suffering and your life experiences.

     a. When you do *not* think, feel, and act like a victim, how do you
        i. think of yourself differently?
        ii. treat yourself differently?
        iii. think and act differently around others?
     b. What conclusions do you draw from this experiment?
     c. What do you see as the pros and cons of applying and living out Frankl's perspective in your daily life?
        i. What are the benefits?
        ii. What are the costs?
        iii. What is scary about this?

IV. Record on the Traumatic Flashback Incident Record flashbacks and nightmares experienced between sessions.

V. Bring homework to next session for review.

SESSION 17

Assess general mood and between-session mood shifts
Review reactions to previous session
Review homework
    Review Traumatic Flashback Incident Record data
    Review and process the written responses to each item of the homework
Continue efforts to create a meaningful cognitive frame for individual suffering
Introduce idea of writing a life narrative
Review safety contract (if applicable)
Assign homework

Allow 90 minutes for session 17. The first few minutes are spent reviewing the patient's general mood, between-session mood shifts, and reactions to the previous session. The therapist briefly inquires about the presence, frequency, and intensity of flashbacks and nightmares since last session, while reviewing the data recorded on the Traumatic Flashback Incident Record.

The focus of the session then shifts to discussing and processing the remainder of the patient's written homework, as the therapist and patient continue their efforts to create a meaningful cognitive frame for the patient's suffering. Specifically, the patient and therapist examine and discuss how other trauma victims have been able to create positive meaning out of their suffering.

The therapist and patient then collaboratively explore how the patient's own traumas might be transformed into meaningful life experiences. Continuing to address the difference between being victimized and viewing oneself as a victim is a critical cognitive component of treatment at this juncture. Even if the patient has made significant progress in mastering traumatic flashbacks, nightmares, and recurring traumatic memories, maintaining an active victimization schema—

continuing to think, feel, and act like a victim—will inhibit further therapeutic progress and growth. Indeed, although the victim may be a survivor of severe childhood trauma, survivors do not become thrivers until they are able to accept their traumatic experiences as part of their lives and transcend their own victimization by finding positive meaning in their suffering. Thus, challenging patients to apply a Frankl-like perspective to their lives and imagining themselves not just as survivors but as thrivers is a critical cognitive component of treatment at this juncture. The ongoing challenge for the therapist during such discussions is to remain supportive of the patient at one level (i.e., communicate empathy and understanding) while firmly confronting the patient's victimization schema at another level.

Patients are also encouraged to engage in dialogue with other trauma survivors and to listen carefully to how others have framed and processed their victimization experiences, the degree to which they have remained stuck in their victimization, how much they have moved beyond victim space and have found meaning in their lives, and the degree to which they have accepted their traumas as part of their history whereby the traumatic experiences are no longer debilitating to them or are a primary focus of their lives. In some instances, it may be useful to explore joining a trauma survivors group, especially if the primary focus is on helping victims to move beyond their victimization. The therapist may suggest additional outside reading about trauma victims who have written about their suffering and their efforts to create meaning out of their lives.

The therapist then introduces the idea of developing a time line, from birth to the present, that includes the patient's major life events and a narrative from the patient's current perspective. It is generally best to present this as an open-ended assignment, so that patients themselves can struggle through the multitude of life experiences they have had and

A HIGHER ORDER COGNITIVE/LINGUISTIC PROCESSING

select the important life events with idiosyncratic meaning to them.

Homework Assignment (Session 17)

I. Write a narrative time line of your life. Include major life events as well as important personal memories. Once you have established the time line, write a brief description of each event, and how this is impacting your current life.

II. Record on the Traumatic Flashback Incident Record flashbacks and nightmares experienced between sessions.

III. Bring homework to next session for review.

SESSION 18

Assess general mood and between-session mood shifts
Review reactions to previous session
Review homework
    Review Traumatic Flashback Incident Record data
    Review narrative
Continue efforts to create a meaningful cognitive frame for individual suffering
Facilitate ADULT–CHILD imagery follow-up
Administer Post-Imagery Questionnaire-B
Process and debrief
Determine if additional imagery sessions are indicated
Address termination (if applicable)
Address need for additional treatment sessions (if applicable)
Review safety contract (if applicable)
Assign homework

Allow 90 minutes for session 18. The first few minutes are spent reviewing the patient's general mood, between-session mood shifts, and reactions to the previous session. The therapist briefly inquires about the presence, frequency, and intensity of flashbacks and nightmares since last session, while reviewing the data recorded on the Traumatic Flashback Incident Record.

The focus of the session then shifts to reviewing the remainder of the written homework, which is the patient's life narrative. The patient is encouraged to read this aloud in the session and may want to pause from time to time to discuss and process various aspects of the narrative with the therapist. As part of this processing, the therapist and patient continue their efforts to create a meaningful cognitive frame for the patient's suffering. Continuing to challenge patients to apply a Frankl-like perspective to their lives and imagining themselves not just as survivors but as thrivers remains a critical cognitive component of this phase of treatment. The therapist continues to gently but firmly confront the patient's maladaptive schemas (e.g., schemas of victimization, unlovability, self-hatred, powerlessness) that may be impeding further progress.

ADULT–CHILD Imagery Follow-Up

The therapist then explains the need for doing a follow-up ADULT–CHILD imagery session to determine whether additional imagery sessions may be indicated. Even though our expectation is that PTSD symptoms abate significantly with this treatment, there are many instances where this amount of treatment alone will not be sufficient to produce a level of adaptive functioning (e.g., interpersonal, occupational, social). In such instances, a longer-term treatment may be indicated. The therapist facilitates the ADULT–CHILD imagery by asking the patient to visually "check in" with the CHILD (as was done in sessions 9 to 13):

> When you are ready, you may close your eyes and visually check in with the CHILD.

The therapist facilitates the imagery follow-up by asking:

> Where is the CHILD?
> What is the CHILD doing?
> How is the CHILD feeling?
> Where are you, the ADULT, in relation to the CHILD?
> How far are you, the ADULT, from the CHILD?
> Does the CHILD see you, the ADULT?
> How does the CHILD respond to your presence?
> How do you, the ADULT, respond to the CHILD's presence?
> How are you, the ADULT, feeling?
> What would you, the ADULT, like to do or say to the CHILD? Can you do/say that to the CHILD directly?
> How does the CHILD respond?
> When you look directly into the CHILD's eyes, what do you see?
> How do you react to what you see in the CHILD's eyes?

Once it appears that the ADULT and CHILD may be ready to end the imagery, the therapist asks:

> Is there anything more that you, the ADULT, would like to do or say to the CHILD before bringing the imagery to a close?

Once the patient has indicated a readiness to terminate the imagery, the therapist responds:

> You may now let the imagery fade away, and when you are ready you may open your eyes.

After the patient has had sufficient time to adapt to the completion of the imagery, the therapist administers the PIQ-B, reading each item aloud to the patient and recording the patient's numerical rating on the line to the left of each item. The therapist again uses the PIQ-B data to obtain immediate patient feedback about the imagery session just experienced, to ascertain overall progress, and to determine if additional imagery sessions might be indicated.

If the patient is able to visualize the ADULT nurturing, comforting, soothing, or interacting comfortably and meaningfully with the CHILD, it is likely that no further imagery sessions are needed at this time. On the other hand, if the patient's ADULT has difficulty nurturing the CHILD or relating meaningfully to the CHILD, or the CHILD appears distant or fearful of letting the ADULT come too close, additional ADULT–CHILD imagery sessions may be indicated. We have observed with this population time and again that patients who continue to struggle with suicidality and self-injurious behaviors have difficulty with the adult-nurturing-child imagery. Again, both the therapist and the patient must collaboratively make the determination of whether additional imagery sessions are indicated at this time.

Addressing Termination (If Applicable)

If it appears that the patient has been able to adequately process (emotionally and cognitively) the childhood traumas and significantly modify maladaptive trauma-related beliefs, attributions, and schemas, the patient may be ready for termination. Specific indicators of the patient's readiness for termination include (1) a significant reduction or elimination of PTSD symptomatology; (2) the absence of further traumatic flashbacks or nightmares; (3) the ability to consistently visualize healthy, self-nurturing imagery; (4) realistic beliefs and attributions of the abuse; (5) the replacement of traumagenic core beliefs/schemas with healthier self-schemas; (6) the ability to accept the traumatic events as part of one's life experience and, if possible, to find positive meaning in one's suffering; (7) ceasing to think, feel, and act like a victim; (8) an enhanced ability to effectively cope with daily stressors; and (9) an absence of self-harming and suicidal behaviors.

If termination is indicated, the therapist and patient review progress made during treatment, identify ongoing stressors in the patient's present life, rehearse coping strategies, and develop a plan for handling possible future crisis situations. The patient is encouraged to engage in self-initiated daily journaling and self-nurturing imagery posttreatment. Since most adult survivors of childhood trauma have a history of considerable difficulty with self-nurturance, patients are urged to continue developing self-nurturing imagery on their own indefinitely, or for as long as they derive benefit from it.

Addressing Additional Treatment Sessions (If Necessary)

If, after going through the eighteen-session program, the patient reports experiencing additional recurring traumatic memories, the clinician and patient may consider additional imagery sessions. In such instances, it is generally best to ask which specific traumatic memory the patient would like to confront and process next. (See treatment format outlined in Chapter 7 for each additional memory.)

By contrast, if the patient no longer experiences recurring traumatic memories, but still has major adjustment difficulties (e.g., suffers from significant anxiety or depression), the clinician may consider using a more standard cognitive-behavioral approach. If, however, the patient continues to engage in self-abusive behaviors, or remains suicidal or parasuicidal, the clinician should consider continuing treatment using a schema-focused, cognitive-behavioral approach that (1) actively identifies and confronts the patient's negative schemas (e.g., schemas of unlovability, inherent badness, defectiveness, mistrust, abandonment); (2) places firm limits on self-abusive, suicidal, or other primitive acting-out behaviors; (3) teaches self-calming/self-soothing strategies; and (4) strongly encourages the patient to continue the search for positive meaning in the traumatic experiences.

Posttreatment Safety Contract (If Necessary)

It is crucial that the patient agrees to a posttreatment safety contract in writing, similar to that which was in effect during treatment. Specifically, the patient agrees

1. not to engage in any self-abusive or self-injurious behaviors, and
2. to implement a mutually agreed upon plan of action (e.g., calling someone, journaling, engaging in a self-calming activity) if feeling strong urges to self-abuse or self-injure.

Posttreatment Guidelines for Crisis Management

The patient may call the therapist if a crisis arises or if serious difficulties are encountered. However, the patient is instructed that the crisis management guidelines in effect since session 8 are still to be followed. Thus, before placing a crisis call to the therapist, the patient is reminded to first visualize and write out an imaginary conversation with the therapist, in which the patient

1. describes the upsetting situation,
2. verbalizes active thoughts and feelings about the situation,
3. describes to the therapist (in imagery) efforts already made to cope with the situation,
4. "listens" carefully to the therapist's response and attentively writes down what she "hears" the therapist saying.

After having this imaginary conversation with the therapist, the patient may call the therapist if she still feels the need to do so. However, the patient understands that upon making such a crisis call, the therapist's initial response will be to ask (1) whether the patient has carried out an imaginary conversation with the therapist, (2) what the patient has written down from that imaginary conversation, and (3) what the patient "saw" and "heard" in the therapist's response.

Homework Assignment (Session 18)

I. Continue working on (writing, revising) your life narrative.

II. Process further your reactions to today's imagery session.
   1. Listen daily to the audiotape of today's imagery session.
   2. Record your SUDs on the Homework Record both prior to and after listening to the audiotaped imagery session.
   3. Fill out the PIQ-B and record the PIQ score on the Homework Record immediately after listening to the audiotaped imagery session.
   4. Write out your personal reactions to the audiotaped imagery session.

III. Visually "check in" daily with the child and engage in self-initiated adult-nurturing-child imagery. Record the experience in a journal.

IV. Record on the Traumatic Flashback Incident Record flashbacks and nightmares experienced.

V. Document efforts to cope with stressful/upsetting situations.

When you find yourself in a stressful/upsetting situation, write down the following:
   1. the upsetting situation and specific stressor;
   2. the specific upsetting thoughts and feelings you have while in the stressful situation;

3. the level of distress felt (on a 1 to 10 scale) immediately before and after efforts to self-calm;
4. how you attempt to self-calm while in the upsetting situation;
5. how you attempt to cope with the situation;
6. how effective your efforts are to self-calm and cope with the upsetting situation;
7. other strategies you might consider when attempting to cope with such stressful situations in the future.

VI. Continue to log daily entries in a journal.

POSTTREATMENT ASSESSMENT

A posttreatment clinical assessment battery, similar to that given at pretreatment, is administered to the patient at the end of the session. If treatment is terminated prior to this session, a posttreatment assessment battery should be given at whatever point treatment ends and again at follow-up.

RELAPSE PREVENTION/MAINTENANCE SESSIONS

Monthly prevention/maintenance sessions are scheduled for as long as they are deemed clinically indicated by both therapist and patient. These follow-up sessions are critical for reinforcing and maintaining gains, as well as for relapse prevention. Allow two hours for each maintenance session.

Administer follow-up assessment battery
Assess general mood and posttreatment mood shifts
Review progress in general
Review entire homework
    Review Traumatic Flashback Incident Record data
    Review additional work on life narrative

A HIGHER ORDER COGNITIVE/LINGUISTIC PROCESSING

    Review efforts to develop self-nurturing imagery and to cope with stressful situations
Facilitate ADULT–CHILD imagery follow-up
Administer Post-Imagery Questionnaire-B
Process and debrief
Review safety contract
Review post-treatment guidelines for crisis management
Assign homework (same homework as in session 18)

We suggest administering the posttreatment follow-up assessment battery after one month, three months, six months, and every six months thereafter for as long as the relapse prevention/maintenance sessions are necessary.

PART III
SPECIAL CONSIDERATIONS

7

Imagery Rescripting Format for Each Additional Recurring Traumatic Memory

SESSION 1 (1.5 HOURS)

Assess general mood
Review homework (if applicable)
Record/review presence and frequency of recurring flashbacks and nightmares on Traumatic Flashback Incident Record
Review efficacy of self-calming/stress-reducing coping strategies
Facilitate imaginal exposure, mastery imagery, and adult-nurturing-child imagery
Administer Post-Imagery Questionnaire-A (PIQ-A)
Process and debrief
Review contract for safety and guidelines for crisis management
Assign homework

SESSION 2 (1.5 HOURS)

Assess general mood
Review homework

> Review presence and frequency of recurring flashbacks and nightmares on Traumatic Flashback Incident Record
> Review reactions to daily audiotape listening
> Review efficacy of self-calming/stress-reducing coping strategies

Facilitate imaginal exposure, mastery imagery, and adult-nurturing-child imagery
Administer Post-Imagery Questionnaire-A (PIQ-A)
Process and debrief
Review contract for safety and guidelines for crisis management
Assign homework

SESSION 3 (1.5 HOURS)

Assess general mood
Review homework
> Review presence and frequency of recurring flashbacks and nightmares on Traumatic Flashback Incident Record
> Review reactions to daily audiotape listening
> Review efficacy of self-calming/stress-reducing coping strategies

Facilitate imaginal exposure, mastery imagery, and adult-nurturing-child imagery
Administer Post-Imagery Questionnaire-A (PIQ-A)
Process and debrief
Determine whether additional exposure and rescripting sessions are indicated
Review contract for safety and guidelines for crisis management
Assign homework

Do not reexperience or rescript traumatic imagery after session 3 unless the ADULT remains unable to confront the perpetrator and rescue the CHILD without difficulty. As a rule, additional exposure/rescripting imagery is indicated if the patient has a score of 50 or greater on item 3 or 4 of the Post-Imagery Questionnaire-A.

SESSION 4 (1.5 HOURS)

Assess general mood
Review homework
    Record/review presence and frequency of flashbacks and nightmares on Traumatic Flashback Incident Record
    Review reactions to daily audiotape listening
    Review efficacy of self-calming/self-soothing strategies
Facilitate adult-nurturing-child imagery
Administer Post-Imagery Questionnaire-B (PIQ-B)
Process and debrief
Review contract for safety and guidelines for crisis management
Assign homework

SESSION 5 (1.5 HOURS)

Assess general mood
Review homework
Record/review presence and frequency of recurring flashbacks and nightmares on Traumatic Flashback Incident Record
Review efficacy of self-calming/self-soothing strategies
Facilitate adult-nurturing-child imagery
Administer Post-Imagery Questionnaire-B (PIQ-B)
Process and debrief
Review progress and determine if additional imagery sessions are indicated

Discuss termination (if applicable)
Review contract for safety and guidelines for crisis management
Assign homework
Administer posttreatment assessment (if applicable)

MONTHLY RELAPSE PREVENTION/MAINTENANCE SESSIONS (2.0 HOURS EACH)

Follow format described in Chapter 6.

Homework Assignment (for Sessions 1–5 and Maintenance/Follow-Up)

 I. Process further your reactions to today's imagery session.

   1. Listen daily to audiotape of the entire imagery session.
   2. Record your SUDs on the Homework Record both prior to and after listening to the audiotaped imagery session.
   3. Fill out the PIQ immediately after listening to the audiotaped imagery session and record the PIQ score on the Homework Record (use the PIQ-A for sessions 1–3, and the PIQ-B for sessions 4–5).
   4. Write out your personal reactions to the audiotaped imagery session in a journal.

 II. Record on the Traumatic Flashback Incident Record flashbacks or nightmares experienced between sessions.

 III. Document efforts to cope with stressful/upsetting situations

   When in an upsetting/stressful situation, write down the following:

   1. the upsetting situation and specific stressor;
   2. the level of distress felt (on a 1 to 10 scale);

3. the specific upsetting thoughts, feelings, and images you have while in the stressful situation;
4. how you attempt to self-calm while in the upsetting situation;
5. how you attempt to cope with the situation;
6. how successful your efforts are to self-calm and cope with the upsetting situation;
7. other strategies you might consider when attempting to cope with such stressful situations in the future.

V. Bring homework to next session for review.

8
When Difficulties Arise during the Imagery Session

If patients for whom imagery rescripting initially seems appropriate experience continued difficulties with the imagery format after several sessions, adaptations to the procedure may need to be implemented. IRRT may need to be suspended for patients who

- engage in significant cognitive avoidance during imagery such that their inability to visually hold or "stay with" a specific traumatic memory or flashback is significantly impeded (e.g., they dissociate repeatedly without being able to respond to the therapist's efforts to keep them focused on the imagery);
- experience significant information overload such that they are repeatedly flooded with intrusive imagery that prevents the implementation of either the exposure or rescripting component of treatment;
- experience significant affective avoidance (e.g., persistent emotional numbing) during exposure or rescripting, which prevents them from reexperiencing and reprocessing the affect.

In such instances, it is sometimes useful to have the patient begin the exposure process by first writing down the traumatic memory in as much detail as possible, followed by making an audiotape of the patient reading it aloud in the therapy session and then asking the patient to listen to the audiotape daily for homework. After several days, the patient may again write down the trauma-related images, thoughts, and feelings, followed by again reading them aloud in the therapy session and listening daily to an audiotape of the session.

If, however, after such efforts the patient continues to experience cognitive or affective avoidance that significantly interferes with the imaginal exposure or rescripting phases, it may be an indication that the patient is feeling too fragile or fragmented to proceed with IRRT at this time, or that the denial/numbing defenses are still necessary to protect the patient from information overload. It may also be that the patient is not feeling trusting enough toward the therapist to engage in this kind of intensive therapeutic work. Although IRRT in such instances may be initially premature, it may be appropriate at some later point in therapy once the patient has developed sufficient trust in the therapeutic relationship and seems in a more overall receptive psychological state (see Chapter 9 for a more extended overview of special treatment options when IRRT is not indicated).

WHEN INSUFFICIENT PROGRESS IS MADE AFTER EIGHT IMAGERY SESSIONS

Significant difficulties may sometimes arise with the more chronically disturbed patients—especially with those who endured severe and prolonged sexual abuse throughout much of their childhood—such that after eight imagery sessions they have not habituated sufficiently to the abuse imagery during exposure or have been unable to develop sufficient empowering/mastery imagery during rescripting. When this occurs, the clinician has several options to consider:

1. Continue with additional exposure and rescripting sessions either with the same abuse memory, or with another relatively less threatening abuse memory following the basic treatment protocol.
2. Progress to ADULT–CHILD imagery sessions. (Clinical experience has shown, however, that ADULT–CHILD imagery is less likely to be successful in such instances.)
3. Suspend imagery sessions and apply more standard behavioral interventions that focus primarily on stress management (e.g., stress inoculation training, relaxation training, focused breathing, grounding techniques).
4. Facilitate a higher order linguistic processing of the abuse memory (or memories) by having the patient write out transcripts of the audiotaped imagery sessions.

While options 1 to 3 are relatively straightforward, option 4 is a cognitive intervention that has not been reported previously in the PTSD literature, but in our experience has been found to be quite successful with highly motivated patients. In the following section, a more detailed description of this intervention is offered.

WRITING OUT AND PROCESSING TRANSCRIPTS OF THE AUDIOTAPED IMAGERY SESSIONS

The therapist introduces the idea of the patient writing or typing transcripts of the first five audiotaped imagery sessions conducted, beginning with that of session 1. The rationale for writing out the imagery transcripts may be explained as follows:

> Some trauma survivors find it useful to write or type out transcripts of the imagery sessions while listening to the audiotape. This involves (1) writing down every word spoken by you and the therapist during all phases of the imagery session; (2) writing down, in parentheses, any other thoughts or feelings you remember having during the imagery; and (3) writing down, in parentheses, thoughts or feelings you have about the abuse as you write out the transcripts. We have learned from other trauma survivors that writing out transcripts of these imagery sessions can help you further emotionally process your traumatic experiences at a verbal level, help you finish working through remaining unprocessed parts of your abuse experience, and help you feel more in control of your flashbacks.
>
> How would you feel about writing out transcripts of session 1 this week as part of your homework? In our next session we would then discuss what the assignment was like for you.

The therapist allows sufficient time to discuss patient reactions to the proposed assignment. The therapist should listen carefully to, understand, and validate any concerns the patient may have, while simultaneously offering the patient reassurance and encouragement to follow through with the assignment. If the patient is agreeable to follow through with this assignment, the therapist may suggest the homework be conducted as follows:

I. Write or type transcripts (in sequence) of the first audiotaped imagery session:

1. Write or type all words spoken by you and the therapist in the imagery sessions. You may use a "T:" in the far left margin to indicate when the therapist is speaking, and a "C:" to indicate when you, the client, are speaking.

2. Write down, in parentheses, as part of the transcripts any thoughts or feelings you remember having during the imagery that you are writing about.
3. Write down, in parentheses, thoughts or feelings you have about the abuse as you write/type the transcripts.

II. Once the transcripts of the first imagery session are completely written or typed, the same procedure (as described above) is followed for the imagery sessions 2 to 5. The number of sessions needed to complete this task is determined by how rapidly the patient is able to complete and process the information adequately.

The therapist and patient will typically spend four to six sessions on writing and processing the transcripts. During each 90-minute transcript-processing session, the written transcripts are read aloud by the patient, discussed, and processed. The therapist begins by asking the patient to share general and journalized reactions to the transcript-writing assignment (e.g., thoughts and feelings about the assignment, how much time it took to complete, how difficult it was, how much dissociation occurred while doing the assignment). The therapist then invites the patient to begin reading the transcripts aloud, beginning with session 1. (It is best if a copy of the transcripts is available so the therapist can follow along while the patient is reading.) From time to time, the patient and therapist will want to pause and discuss, or further process, portions of the transcripts, especially those parts to which the patient still responds with relatively heightened affect. It is important that the patient read aloud, in the presence of the therapist, all five session transcripts, a process that often takes several therapy sessions to complete.

With some patients it may be useful, and even essential, to read, discuss, and process the transcripts a second time with the therapist. (This decision should be made collaboratively by the patient and therapist.) In such instances, the therapist will want to ascertain the relative degree of distress that the patient experiences while reading through the transcripts the second time, how much dissociation occurs while reading and processing the transcripts, and what effect the transcript-writing/linguistic processing of the imagery sessions is having on the presence, frequency, and intensity of the traumatic memories themselves. Once again, the patient and therapist will, from time to time, want to pause and process specific portions of the transcripts, especially those parts that may still trigger heightened affect.

After completion of the transcript-writing and processing sessions, it is best to return to and follow the session 7 imagery format, which involves the reexperiencing (exposure) and rescripting of the traumatic imagery. If the patient has sufficiently habituated (during exposure) and rescripted the abuse imagery (i.e., has a score of less than 50 on items 2 and 3 of the Post-Imagery Questionnaire-A), then treatment may proceed to session 8 and the ADULT–CHILD only imagery format.

9

When Imagery Rescripting Is Not Indicated: Alternate Cognitive-Behavioral Treatment Options

TREATING PARTIAL PTSD-RELATED SYMPTOMS

Trauma-related, PTSD-like symptoms frequently observed among treatment-seeking adult survivors of childhood trauma, for whom IRRT may not be initially indicated, tend to comprise the following areas: increased arousal, generalized emotional numbing, dissociation, and partial intrusive ideation. This chapter discusses each of these traumagenic symptom areas, and offers guidelines for their conceptualization and initial treatment considerations within a cognitive-behavioral therapy context (Smucker 1997).

Increased Arousal

Some adult patients report clinical symptoms of increased arousal to be the most prominent and distressing (e.g., hypervigilance, exaggerated startle response, generalized fear/anxiety). Such responses may be partial manifestations of a PTSD syndrome not yet fully activated that serve to block out (cognitive avoidance) intrusive traumatic memories, visual flashbacks, and associated affect. In the case of PTSD, such increased arousal symptoms may indeed serve to keep specific trauma-related stimuli outside of one's conscious level of awareness. Such individuals may present as extremely anxious, fearful, tense, rigid, and unable to relax as they appear to be constantly scanning the horizon waiting for the "next bomb to drop" (Smucker 1997).

On the other hand, increased arousal symptoms in and of themselves do not necessarily indicate the presence of an underlying PTSD syndrome. Such symptoms could reflect the presence of other non-PTSD clinical phenomena, such as generalized anxiety, acute stress, phobic avoidance, agoraphobia, or schema-driven anxiety (e.g., abandonment panic). In such instances, a more standard form of anxiety-management treatment might be indicated (e.g., stress inoculation training).

As is customary with most forms of cognitive-behavioral therapy, the initial focus of treatment is on identifying the specific problems for which the patient is seeking help, followed by establishing mutually agreed upon goals that are specific and realistic in nature. If a treatment goal is to eliminate or significantly reduce the increased arousal symptoms, both therapist and patient should understand that working toward this goal could lead to a short-term exacerbation of involuntary, intrusive traumatic images and associated painful affect. At the same time, the emergence of such symptoms may provide a therapeutic opportunity that facilitates and enhances emotional processing of the traumatic material, and thus be beneficial to the patient's long-term recovery. Should the patient react negatively or with hesitation to this caveat, it may be useful to conduct a collaborative cost-benefit analysis weighing the pros and cons (short-term and long-term) of confronting and working through the PTSD symptomatology versus maintaining the current status quo.

If the patient decides that reducing the increased arousal symptoms is a desirable treatment goal, even if it leads to the activation of other posttraumatic stress symptoms, a multipronged cognitive-behavioral approach may be used that involves identifying and challenging the beliefs and schemata underlying the increased arousal symptoms (e.g., schemas of vulnerability, powerlessness, mistrust), while simultaneously helping the patient develop more adaptive behavioral coping strategies for daily functioning. Specifically, the clinician may utilize a schema-focused approach (Young 1994), together with more traditional cognitive therapy (Leahy 1996) and stress inoculation training interventions (e.g., monitoring mood and activities, graded task assignments, relaxation training, focused breathing, self-calming imagery training, skills acquisition training, grounding techniques, increasing physical exercise, and overall physical activity). (See Foa and colleagues [1991] and Meichenbaum [1993] for a detailed description of stress inoculation training.) Mood-stabilizing psychiatric medications may also be employed as part of treatment.

In instances where patients appear too psychologically fragile, are too fearful of change, do not feel trusting enough of the therapist, or are not yet ready to give up their defenses, it is sometimes better to begin less ambitiously by combining psychopharmacology with a more supportive approach that focuses on affective stabilization and trust building. With some severely traumatized patients, a solid therapeutic alliance must often first be in place before IRRT or other cognitive-behavioral interventions can be effectively employed.

Generalized Emotional Numbing

Some victims of multiple and prolonged childhood traumas attempt to escape and avoid all trauma-related pain by completely shutting down emotionally. These individuals are terrified that they will be overwhelmed and totally consumed by their pain if they allow themselves to feel anything at all.

While perhaps offering some temporary, short-term protection from feeling overwhelmed by painful emotions, such affective avoidance strategies do not rescue trauma survivors from their *mal de vivre*, but rather keep them stuck in their traumatization, prevent them from experiencing the range of normal human emotions, and result in a lonely existence devoid of human intimacy and interpersonal bonding.

Once again, it is important to clarify the specific problem areas for which help is being sought, as well as specific treatment goals, before beginning treatment. If the patient's stated therapeutic goal is to become emotionally alive and to be able to feel again—in short, to be able to experience affect of any kind for longer periods of time—it may be important for the clinician to understand why and how the patient has come to that decision. Although survivors may understand the likely long-term benefits of such therapeutic work, they must also understand that opening themselves up to their feelings may, in the short term, activate intense negative emotions, unleash painful traumatic memories, and/or even lead to a full-blown PTSD response.

If the patient is motivated nonetheless to move ahead toward emotional de-numbing, any number of affective-regulation skill-building exercises could be implemented (both in and out of the therapy session) that focus on increasing affective tolerance (Briere 1992). The clinician will need to emphasize again and again that feelings are only feelings, that feelings in and of themselves are not dangerous and are not harbingers of impending harm, and that one can become desensitized to—and eventually integrate—traumatic memories and emotions without resorting to primitive defenses that thwart adequate emotional processing. At the same time, it is critical that the clinician be sensitive to the patient's overall emotional state, psychological fragility, fear of change, and likely feelings of mistrust vis-à-vis the therapist.

The clinician must also consider the possibility that further exposure to traumatic material may at times exceed the survivor's internal resources and capacity for affect regulation. If indeed the trauma survivor's psychological defenses appear to be crumbling and the individual is beginning to feel overwhelmed with the emergence of heightened painful affect, clarifying the specific treatment goals becomes the primary and most essential therapeutic task. If, for example, the patient is seeking the therapist's help in developing better affective avoidance strategies, the therapist may initially normalize the survivor's need to self-protect—especially from feeling overwhelmed by emotional pain—but also explain how trauma victims tend to remain stuck when they attempt to numb themselves to or bury their emotions, that emotional processing of traumatic events is critical to recovery, and that survivors can only get beyond their pain by going through it. Above all, it is important for trauma survivors to understand that while emotional pain is unavoidable, they do have a choice of opting either for pain that leads to recovery (growing pains) or for pain that keeps them stuck (stagnation pains).

Here again, it may be necessary to begin treatment with a less ambitious therapeutic posture, for example, employing pharmacological interventions for initial mood stabilization and a relatively noninterventionistic/supportive therapeutic approach that focuses on affective stabilization, trust building, and the development of a therapeutic alliance, before attempting to implement IRRT or other cognitive-behavioral interventions. Regardless of what phase of treatment trauma survivors are in, therapy with this population is most effective when applied within the context of clearly defined treatment goals.

Dissociation

The presence of frequent dissociative episodes sometimes emerges as a prominent and distressing clinical symptom of trauma survivors. While dissociation often appears to function as an "affective anesthetic" by shielding individuals from painful trauma-related stimuli and providing an escape from unpleasant affect associated with the pressures and stress of the moment, for adults it is a relatively primitive response that can be quite dysfunctional, produce a state of psychological regression, interfere with productive functioning at work and at home, and lead to aversive consequences. Frequent dissociation can put individuals at risk for losing their job or partner because the boss or partner may lose patience and no longer be willing to put up with their dissociative episodes and unproductivity. As noted by Briere (1992), "Dissociation and primitive tension-reduction activities can be maladaptive or injurious by virtue of their inherent properties (e.g., drug abuse or indiscriminate sex) or because of their tendency to reduce the survivor's accurate responsiveness to environmental demands" (p. 120).

The initial treatment focus with dissociative individuals is to educate them about the nature and function of dissociation, emphasizing both its adaptive and maladaptive aspects. The clinician and patient then conduct a collaborative assessment on the costs and benefits of the continued use of dissociation as a coping strategy. It is important that individuals fully understand the maladaptive effects that dissociation has on their overall level of functioning, and that the benefits of dissociation are at best a short-lived escape from immediate emotional pain. Patients also need to understand that a likely short-term cost of not dissociating is to experience periodic waves of intense and painful emotions that may at times feel unbearable.

If a patient is not yet ready to give up dissociation as a coping strategy, a less ambitious therapeutic approach may be preferable, one that combines psychiatric medication with a more supportive approach that focuses on trust building, affective stabilization, and affect-regulation skill building (Briere 1992).

By contrast, when patients appear sufficiently motivated to give up their dissociation defenses, a more ambitious cognitive-behavioral intervention program may be implemented, with the focus on developing alternate coping strategies to replace the dissociation episodes while simultaneously developing strategies to increase the patient's tolerance for emotional pain. If the therapy goals are thus to significantly reduce or eliminate all dissociative episodes and to increase the patient's tolerance for emotional pain, an array of cognitive-behavioral interventions may be utilized on a trial-and-error basis (e.g., affective tolerance training, stress inoculation training, prolonged exposure, relaxation training, focused breathing), together with psychopharmacological treatment.

Partial Intrusive Ideation

Some traumatized patients report the presence of partial trauma-related memories/flashbacks, as they appear to oscillate between PTSD-like intrusions and denial/numbing responses. In some such instances, patients may still be blocking out painful parts of their traumatic memories. To facilitate activation of the entire traumatic fear network, prolonged imaginal exposure may be considered. However, the clinician must proceed very cautiously with any interventions when patients report partial, vague, or nebulous memories of traumatic events and, above all, refrain from being suggestive or engaging in memory reconstruction or the creation of false memories.

PART IV
CASE STUDIES

10

Case Example 1: One-Session IRRT

One of the first imagery rescripting cases the senior author was asked to work with was Mary, a 40-year-old inpatient who had been raped at age 19 (by the grandfather of the children she was babysitting) and who had subsequently experienced recurring traumatic nightmares several times per week for the next twenty-one years. In addition to suffering from PTSD, Mary was experiencing chronic sleep disturbance as well as generalized anxiety and depression. The referring psychiatrist asked for a one-session cognitive therapy treatment consult to determine whether cognitive therapy could be useful in helping to eliminate this twenty-one-year recurring nightmare.

During the subsequent consultation session with Mary, she related experiencing a recurring nightmare two to three times weekly for twenty-one years—the same nightmare each time in its original form, exactly how she had remembered experiencing the sexual assault itself at age 19—and that each time she had the nightmare she felt "violated and raped all over again." In spite of many years in psychiatric treatment, Mary reported receiving no help with her repetitive nightmares.

Conceptualizing her affective distress within a cognitive framework brought to the fore one of the most basic tenets of the cognitive therapy model: that emotional pain is directly linked to negative/upsetting cognitions, and that modifying one's upsetting cognitions has been empirically demonstrated to significantly alleviate the associated affective distress. The target "hot" cognitions in Mary's case appeared to be the recurring victimization imagery embedded in her recurring nightmare. Underlying her repetitive nightmare images of sexual victimization and helplessness vis-à-vis the perpetrator appeared to be a schema of powerlessness. It begged the question: If Mary were able to "contaminate" and replace the rape-related victimization imagery with empowering/mastery imagery in the office—e.g., visualizing herself overpowering and subduing the perpetrator—might she then be able to take these rescripted mastery images with her from the session and modify the victimization imagery in her nightmare as well, perhaps even eliminate her terrifying nightmares?

During the consult, Mary was asked if she would be willing to do some imagery work with the nightmare. She readily agreed, noting that she had been haunted by this terrifying nightmare for over half of her life and was therefore willing to try almost anything. Mary was then asked to close her eyes and visualize the beginning of the nightmare, verbalizing aloud what she experienced. Mary was able to vividly visualize and verbalize the entire nightmare/sexual assault scene along with a great deal of affective distress.

After Mary completed her verbal description and affective reliving of the entire nightmare, she was asked to again visualize and verbalize the sexual assault scene from the beginning. This time through, however, when Mary began to describe the actual rape imagery of the nightmare, she was asked what she might want to do differently. She replied that she'd like to kick him (the perpetrator) hard in the crotch. Mary was then asked if she could, at that moment, visualize herself kicking him as hard as she could in the crotch, which she was readily able to do. When asked how he was responding to her kick, Mary replied: "He's lying on the floor, screaming out in pain... and he deserves it." This became an empowering moment for Mary as she proceeded, in imagery, to kick him a few more times. Mary was then able to visualize herself expressing directly to the perpetrator her thoughts and feelings about the abuse (something that she had not been able to verbalize previously) and that it was now his turn to suffer.

By the end of the imagery session, Mary's affect had shifted dramatically. She was not only smiling, but appeared empowered and elated. Upon leaving the office a few minutes later, however, she became visibly upset at the thought of having the nightmare again that night, which she said occurred whenever she spoke to anyone about it. Mary was then asked if she wouldn't like to "get him really good one more time," to which she responded by smiling and saying, "Yes, I would. I guess I just wasn't thinking about it in that way." The following morning when the therapist entered the inpatient unit, Mary approached him with a big smile on her face and said, "Dr. Smucker, he came back last night and I got him really good!" She cheerfully reported how she had overpowered the perpetrator in her nightmare just as she had done in the imagery session the previous day.

Although no further therapy sessions with Mary were held, the therapist followed up with her by phone on a regular basis after that to inquire whether she had had any more nightmares. With each contact, Mary reported a continued absence of nightmares. The last follow-up contact with Mary was six months after the rescripting session, at which point she continued to be completely free of nightmares.

While this was an unusually short-term use of imagery rescripting interventions with a PTSD patient, it seemed to make sense theoretically that such drastic change could happen so quickly, especially with a type I trauma. (To be sure, such a rapid cognitive shift would not be expected with a recurring abuse memory resulting from a type II trauma.) In short, when the upsetting, rape-related victimization images embedded in her recurring nightmare were activated, confronted, and replaced with empowering imagery, within the context of a therapeutic secure base, Mary was able to internalize and summon up these new mastery images in her nightmare that night and thereby eliminate her terrifying, twenty-one-year nightmare.

While Mary and her treatment team were very pleased with her dramatic turnaround after just one imagery rescripting session, a number of titillating questions remained:

- Did Mary have the capability all along of modifying and stopping the nightmare?
- Could she have been spared the previous twenty-one years of being haunted by this terrifying nightmare if a similar intervention had been implemented earlier in her treatment?
- Had Mary's previous psychiatric treatments failed because they reinforced (inadvertently) her sense of helplessness by not focusing on teaching her how to empower herself?
- Do other abuse victims also have the power within themselves to recover from debilitating posttraumatic symptoms as Mary did?
- Was it, above all, our task as clinicians to help trauma victims recognize and access their own inner psychological resources and self-healing powers?

Grappling with these and other such questions helped to lay the theoretical groundwork and conceptual foundation of IRRT. In short, it was Mary's dramatic and rapid recovery from her twenty-one-year recurring nightmare that became a major impetus and inspiration for the authors in the development of IRRT with traumatized patients suffering from PTSD, especially with adults experiencing recurring flashbacks of their childhood abuse traumas.

11

Case Example 2: Eight-Session IRRT[1]

---

1. This case has been described elsewhere (Smucker and Niederee 1995).

Sarah, a 39-year-old, married, Caucasian woman, is a survivor of childhood sexual abuse. She was referred by her primary therapist (who was not trained to work with PTSD) for IRRT because of recurrent, debilitating flashbacks. She had developed PTSD symptoms four years earlier when her daughter was 3 years old, the age at which she herself had first been molested. Sarah reported a history of sexual abuse perpetrated by her father beginning when she was 3 and lasting until she was 16, ranging from fondling to oral sex and violent rape. Throughout much of her adolescence and adulthood she was chronically depressed, frequently suicidal, anorexic, prone to panic attacks during physical examinations, and was hospitalized on four occasions.

At the time of her referral for IRRT, Sarah met *DSM-IV* criteria for PTSD and suffered from severe depression and a pervasive sense of hopelessness. She reported experiencing debilitating abuse flashbacks daily for several months prior to her first imagery rescripting session. In the wake of each intrusive memory, she reported feeling "betrayed, shameful, guilty, confused, angry, fragmented, and despairing." Sarah's abuse-related cognitions included viewing herself as "vulnerable, powerless, rejected, alone, and hopeless." Thus, alleviation of PTSD symptoms as well as modification of traumagenic core beliefs/schemas were the goals for Sarah's treatment.

COURSE OF IMAGERY RESCRIPTING

The shorter imagery rescripting format (Smucker et al. 1995) was used with Sarah, which consisted of eight imagery sessions only. It omitted the higher order cognitive/linguistic processing component.

During the first three imagery sessions, schemas of powerlessness, abandonment, and mistrust emerged. As the helplessness/powerlessness schema was confronted and weakened, Sarah began to develop a sense of personal empowerment and efficacy. By the fifth session, the helplessness/powerlessness schema no longer appeared dominant. As subsequent sessions focused solely on ADULT–CHILD interactions, a different set of pathogenic beliefs began to surface (e.g., worthlessness, self-blame, inherent badness). The seventh session illustrates the ways in which such schemas are manifested in the ADULT–CHILD dialogue, and how they can be confronted and modified during imagery. The following interchanges are taken from Sarah's first, third, and seventh imagery sessions.

Session 1

After determining the focus of intervention to be Sarah's most debilitating flashback (a recurrent flashback of Sarah's father raping her at age 8) the therapist began the exposure phase of imagery work (reexperiencing the flashback).

> *Therapist:* When you are ready, you may close your eyes and visualize the very beginning of the abuse scene. When you have a clear picture of the abuse, you may

begin to describe aloud what you are experiencing, in the present tense, as though it's happening right now.

Client: I'm in my bedroom getting ready to fall asleep, but I'm feeling really scared and apprehensive. I hear my father starting to come down the hallway. He comes into the bedroom and closes the door. He comes over to the bed, and he starts to unbutton my shirt. I'm pretending I'm asleep but it really doesn't do any good. . . . And then he starts to touch my breasts and fondle them. And (voice becomes shaky) I'm trying to ignore it. I just freeze.

Sarah continues to describe the abuse memory, which ended in her being raped. She attempted to cope with the experience through dissociation.

Client: And all I know is that it hurts a lot. . . . And I can't really see anything, except I focus on the neighbor's kitchen light. . . . So I just go there, go into the light, and try to stay there till it's over. And it seems like it's forever. And then finally, he's done, and . . . just leaves.
Therapist: How are you feeling at this moment?
Client: In some ways . . . I'm glad it's over, I'm just relieved, glad I got through that. But I'm feeling dirty (pause) and messed up.
Therapist: And what's happening now?
Client: Well, I try to pull myself together . . . curl up in a little ball, and put the blanket over me, and try to go to sleep. But I'm feeling abandoned, and I want my mom. And even though I don't really call out for her, it's like I want to. But I know she's not going to be there for me. So I just . . . try to go to sleep . . . and just push it all out of my mind.

With the exposure component of the session completed, the focus then shifted to rescripting the abuse scene. During exposure, Sarah accessed the visual, verbal, and affective components of her experience, revealing schemas of powerlessness, mistrust, and abandonment. During the rescripting phase that follows, her traumagenic schemas are clarified and challenged through imaginal action and dialogue. Initially, her powerlessness schema is confronted, as illustrated in the following segment.

> *Therapist:* I'd like you now to go back to the very beginning of the abuse scene and start to verbalize the abuse as you experienced it. At some point I will assist you in changing the imagery to create a better outcome, one that leaves you feeling more empowered and in control. When you are ready, you may visualize the beginning of the abuse scene and once again describe what is happening to you, in the present tense.

Sarah again describes the abuse imagery, but this time as she begins to reexperience the molestation the therapist facilitates the rescripting process (i.e., the development of mastery imagery) with a prompted transformation.

> *Therapist:* Can you now, at this moment, visualize yourself as an adult today entering the scene, coming into the room? Can you get a picture of that?
> *Client:* Yeah.
> *Therapist:* Where are you, the ADULT, in relation to the CHILD?
> *Client:* I'm standing by the door.
> *Therapist:* What would you, the ADULT, like to do at this point?
> *Client:* I'd like to find a way to get him out of the room, but he's bigger than I am.
> *Therapist:* You'd like to find a way to get him out of the room, but he's bigger than you are. How would you like to get him out of the room?

Client: Well, he's startled, like everything he had done had been kept in secret. So I just say, "What are you doing?" (voice raised, strident). It seems like he's always fearful of being found out.

Therapist: So he doesn't want to be found out. He likes to do things in secret. So you yell out, "What are you doing here?"

Client: Yeah.

Therapist: And how does he respond?

Client: He seems shaken, but it's like he's saying, "I'm not doing anything."

Therapist: And how do you respond?

Client: I say, "Yes you are. Get out of here and leave her alone."

Therapist: And how does he respond?

Client: He tries to get up off the bed... looks at me really mean, like he's trying to scare me.

Therapist: So he gets up... looks at you in a mean way, trying to scare you. And how would you like to respond?

Client: Look him straight in the eye, and say, "Get out of here!"

Therapist: Can you look him in the eyes and tell him to get out?

Client: Yes.

Therapist: And how does he react?

Client: He comes across the room and threatens me, but he doesn't do anything. He just says, "I'll get you later," and pushes at my shoulders to get me off balance. But he can't really hurt me.

Therapist: And what happens at this point?

Client: Then he just leaves. He turns off the light and goes.

Activating her ADULT self in the rescripting process enables Sarah to take a crucial first step in confronting her powerlessness schema—to redefine herself as an autonomous adult capable of taking action to terminate a traumatic event and preserve her own integrity. This newfound sense of efficacy presents a sharp contrast to the pervasive helplessness and paralysis experienced by the CHILD, as illustrated during the self-nurturing phase. In the segment that follows, the ADULT responds to the paralyzed CHILD.

Therapist: So he's gone now, and he turned off the light. And what's happening to the CHILD?
Client: She's just sitting there, kind of frozen.
Therapist: She's sitting there, like she's frozen?
Client: Lying down, frozen.
Therapist: And would you like to react to the CHILD?
Client: I go over to the bed, and I say, "I'm here, and I'm going to protect you." But she's still frozen. And she has tears in her eyes.
Therapist: She's still frozen but she starts to cry. And how do you, the ADULT, respond to her tears?
Client: I say it's okay to cry, but I don't want to touch her. I'm afraid I might startle her. I'd like to hug her but I'm afraid that will scare her.
Therapist: Do you want to ask her if it's okay to hug her?
Client: I think I'll ask her if she wants to sit up.
Therapist: Okay. And how does she respond?
Client: She just sort of sits up and starts to button her pajamas and put the bottoms back on.
Therapist: And how is she feeling right now?
Client: She feels safer, because somebody knows.

Sarah then describes her struggle to take the CHILD from the house to a safe place. Her actions are tentative, and she is momentarily blocked by her mother, who forbids them to leave the family. She is able, however, to take "Little Sarah" to the car and escape. As she and the CHILD are leaving, Sarah states:

> *Client:* I think my anger is helping me to get into the car and drive away. And the little girl is kind of in shock. She didn't think I'd do anything to help her.
> *Therapist:* She didn't really expect anyone to help her?
> *Client:* She didn't expect it—she thought she was stuck there. She thought there was no way out.

Sarah is beginning to establish a bond between her CHILD and ADULT. The ADULT is able to nurture the CHILD by sharing her pain and her story. In Sarah's words, "She feels safer because somebody knows."

Session 3

In the rescripting phase of the third session, Sarah visualizes herself being challenged by her father, who initially refuses to leave the room. Only when she allows herself to become angry and to "not back off" is she able to perceive herself as powerful and able to overcome his intimidation.

> *Therapist:* So you feel yourself getting bigger as you get angrier. Bigger and less afraid. And what's happening now?
> *Client:* I don't back off. I just really yell, "Get out of here!" I'm angry, letting him know that I'm not scared.
> *Therapist:* And when you yell really loud for him to get out of there, how does he respond?
> *Client:* He's having trouble getting up, but he gets up and leaves.

This sense of personal control and efficacy generalizes to her child images as well. Little Sarah is no longer "frozen" in a powerless state of victimization; when her father leaves the room she immediately moves toward the ADULT and asks to leave with her.

In the imagery that follows, the ADULT Sarah challenges a negative injunction from her mother and takes direct action to escape from her former "stuck" position. Through subsequent rescripting, Sarah is able to create a nurturing, protecting adult role model for her CHILD—something she never had as a child.

> *Client:* Little Sarah wants to go with me. She sees me as, not more powerful really, but as someone who will protect her. So I say, "We'd better get out of here. Do you want to come with me?" And she says, "Yes." And so I take her by the hand and get her out of the bed. We start to go through the bedroom and down the hallway, and there's Mom. And Mom's protesting, saying, "You can't leave. Nobody leaves this family."
>
> *Therapist:* And how do you respond to that?
>
> *Client:* I just say that I'm not responsible for her, and I'm taking the little girl with me and leaving.
>
> *Therapist:* And where do you go with her?
>
> *Client:* Out the front door . . . to my car . . . to the place where I live now.
>
> *Therapist:* And how is the CHILD responding to you?
>
> *Client:* She keeps saying in her mind, "This person stood up to my father, and won." And she thinks the ADULT wasn't afraid of her dad. And she's kind of in awe of someone that could stand up to her dad.
>
> *Therapist:* That someone stood up to him and actually won.
>
> *Client:* And didn't seem afraid. So she doesn't seem as afraid.

The above excerpts illustrate successive modifications of trauma-based schemas. Sarah's perception of herself as a powerless, frozen victim is being altered and replaced with a sense of empowerment; she is becoming an active agent, able to bring about change and protect herself from harm. A sense of safety begins to replace chronic mistrust as the ADULT consistently rescues the CHILD from harm and provides a secure environment. By the fifth session, Sarah's flashbacks of this abuse experience have ceased, and subsequent imagery focuses solely on nurturing the CHILD. It is at this point that core beliefs of self-hatred, self-blame, and unlovability begin to emerge in the ADULT–CHILD interactions.

Session 7

Before beginning the imagery work in this session, Sarah discusses difficulties she encountered while listening to her homework tapes. She reports becoming distraught when attempting to nurture the CHILD, stating that she was "not at all accustomed to nurturance" and found it extremely distressing "because it's going against self-hatred." In attempting to articulate her feelings she noted, "It's like I'm holding that child responsible, like it's her fault. Almost like I want to punish her, not nurture her, because it's her fault I was abused." Such themes pervade the early stages of session 7.

> *Therapist:* When you're ready you may close your eyes and get a mental picture of the CHILD. Where is she, what is she doing, how is she feeling?
> *Client:* The CHILD is hiding in an attic.
> *Therapist:* The CHILD is hiding in an attic? Why is she hiding in an attic?
> *Client:* Because she's feeling bad.
> *Therapist:* She's feeling bad. What is she feeling bad about?
> *Client:* She, um, is by herself, she just hates herself.
> *Therapist:* She hates herself. Where are you in the imagery?
> *Client:* Outside of the attic.
> *Therapist:* And what would you, the ADULT, like to do at this point?
> *Client:* Shut the door and lock her in there.

Therapist: What if you shut the door and locked her in there, what would be the effect of that? How would that affect the CHILD?

Client: She'll be closed off... locked away. I could just forget about her.

Therapist: And how will that be for the CHILD?

Client: Terrifying.

Therapist: Terrifying. Do you want the CHILD to be terrified, to be locked away and have a terrifying experience? Is that what you're saying?

Client: I don't want her to be afraid, I just want her to go away.

Therapist: Would you be able to say that to her, to the CHILD directly?

Client: I think so.

Therapist: Would you be open to going up to her in the attic and telling her this—telling her what you are going to do or what you would like to do?

Client: Yeah, I can do it.

On several occasions during this phase of the imagery, Sarah is asked to move closer to the CHILD, to look into her eyes, and talk directly to her. (It appears that trauma-based self-schemas of unlovability and self-hatred can be more effectively activated and challenged when the ADULT is able to gain direct access to the CHILD's pain, perceptions, and frame of reference.) Indeed, as Sarah the ADULT moves closer in proximity to Sarah the CHILD, the ADULT becomes affected by the CHILD's pain and finds it more difficult to continue blaming, hurting, or abandoning the CHILD. As a result, Sarah is now able, for the first time, to place the responsibility for the abuse on the perpetrator.

Therapist: Can you get a picture now of you, the ADULT, going into the attic and going up to the little girl?

Client: Yeah. I go up to the door and look in and say, "I'm going to lock you in here. I'm going to shut the door, I'm not going to let you out."

Therapist: And how does the CHILD respond?

Client: She says, "Please don't lock me in here."

Therapist: How close are you to the CHILD?

Client: I'm still pretty far away, like in a corner, ten feet away.

At this point the therapist asks Sarah to move closer to the CHILD, look into her eyes, and talk to her directly.

Client: (to CHILD) "I'm tired of you being here, I don't want to hear from you, and I want to lock you away in this attic. And I just want you to stay here until you die." (voice very flat and hard).

Therapist: Are you still looking directly into her eyes?

Client: (Nods).

Therapist: And how does the CHILD respond as she looks back up at you?

Client: She says, "Please don't abandon me in here."

Therapist: What do you, the ADULT, see in her eyes as she says that?

Client: Fear.

Therapist: Fear? She's pleading with you not to abandon her?

Client: She's afraid, and she feels self-hatred too.

Therapist: And how do you respond when she says, "Please don't abandon me?"

Client: "I don't want any part of you, it's your fault."

It is often necessary for the ADULT to first express anger and blame to the CHILD directly before core beliefs of self-blame and self-hatred can be effectively challenged and modified.

Therapist: And how does the 5-year-old respond?

Client: "I know it's my fault, but I don't want to be left alone."

Therapist: How close are you to the CHILD at this moment?

Client: I'm still an arm's length away.

Therapist: So the CHILD says to you that she knows it was her fault, but she still doesn't want to be left alone? And how do you respond?

Client: "I just can't have you be a part of my life, you'll just mess it all up."

Therapist: Are you looking at her directly in the eyes as you say that?

Client: I am, but now I'm starting to feel bad about what I see in her eyes.

Therapist: You feel bad about what you see in her eyes? What do you see in her eyes that you're feeling bad about?

Client: She hurts.

Therapist: You see her hurting. And why does that make you feel bad?

Client: Because I decided I didn't want to hurt anyone else the way I was hurt as a child. That was wrong.

Therapist: You decided you never wanted to hurt anyone else the way you were hurt as a child. And here you are, hurting this little child?

Client: Yeah. I'm doing exactly what I said I would never do.

Therapist: Can you attempt to put some of this into words to the child? Can you say that to her directly?

Client: "I don't want to hurt you." It feels like I'm still saying a lie though. Somehow it's still okay for me to hurt her.

Therapist: Can you say that to her directly, perhaps moving a bit closer to her?

Client: "It's okay for me to hurt you because you're the only person I can hurt."

Therapist: And how does the CHILD respond?

Client: It's not okay.

Therapist: The CHILD says it's not okay. Does she say why it's not okay?
Client: I don't know.
Therapist: Can you ask her? Would you like to know why it's not okay?
Client: "Why is it not okay that I hurt you? After all, it's your fault."
Therapist: And how does the CHILD respond?
Client: "What's my fault?"
Therapist: And how do you respond?
Client: "You did terrible things with your father."
Therapist: And how does the CHILD respond?
Client: "I did what Daddy told me to do."
Therapist: And how do you, the ADULT, respond?
Client: "You could have stopped him."
Therapist: And how does the CHILD respond?
Client: "I love my daddy and I want to do what he tells me to do. I want him to love me."
Therapist: So she says she loved her daddy and always wanted to do what he told her to do. And how do you, the ADULT, respond?
Client: "You should have hated him."
Therapist: And how does the CHILD respond?
Client: "Daddy's not bad, I can't hate him."
Therapist: "Daddy's not bad, I can't hate him," she says. And how do you, the ADULT, respond?
Client: I don't want to talk with her anymore.

In the foregoing ADULT–CHILD interaction, Sarah articulated the "abuse dichotomy" (Briere 1989) common to survivors of childhood sexual abuse: if the father is not evil, then the child must be. The following segment illustrates the use of Socratic imagery to facilitate resolution of this dilemma.

Therapist: You don't want to talk with her anymore. Can you tell her that directly?
Client: "I don't want to talk with you anymore."

Therapist: How close are you to her right now?
Client: I backed up.
Therapist: How far away are you?
Client: About five feet.
Therapist: Can you move up close to her again, look her in the eyes, and say that to her?
Client: (long pause) If I get close, I feel confronted with the truth.
Therapist: And what is the truth?
Client: That she's just a little child and she doesn't understand.
Therapist: The truth is, she's just a little child and she doesn't understand. But when you back off from her?
Client: I don't have to face it.
Therapist: You don't have to face the truth?
Client: The truth is, she was little and just did what he said. She didn't have adult reasoning.
Therapist: She was just a child and didn't have adult reasoning?
Client: She didn't realize my father was the bad one.
Therapist: Because she didn't know her father was the bad one, she didn't fight him off. So when you're close up to her and you're talking to her, when you're right next to her, you say you see the truth. But when you back off and move away, that's when you don't see the truth? Or what happens when you back off like that?
Client: If I back off I don't have to deal with it.
Therapist: You don't have to deal with the truth?
Client: Just cut it off or compartmentalize it someplace else. It's like she doesn't exist if I don't think about it.
Therapist: What is it about dealing with the truth that is so difficult for you?
Client: That ... I've spent my whole life blaming that little girl.

Sarah's schema of self-blame and inherent badness is thus identified and called into question. She now begins to denigrate herself for having hated the child, thus placing the blame upon herself as an adult rather than upon herself as a child. In subsequent dialogue, Sarah acknowledges her long-standing fear since childhood of directing her anger toward the primary source of her distress and placing responsibility appropriately upon the perpetrator. The application of Socratic imagery is again illustrated to facilitate resolution of this dilemma.

>   *Therapist:* It sounds like you either have to hate the CHILD or hate yourself for having hated the CHILD? Is that what you're saying?
>   *Client:* That's what I'm saying.
>   *Therapist:* So what is a way out of this dilemma?
>   *Client:* To find some other way of getting rid of the hate.
>   *Therapist:* And what other way might there be to get rid of the hate?
>   *Client:* To finally acknowledge that it's really my father that I hate.
>   *Therapist:* Are you saying that perhaps you've never done that?
>   *Client:* I've been afraid to.
>   *Therapist:* You've been afraid to. Just like the little child was afraid to when her father was doing these things to her. You, as an adult today, are still afraid to, is that what you're saying?
>   *Client:* Yeah.
>   *Therapist:* As a child you continued to see your father as a good person, even when he was doing all these terrible things to you. What do you think about that?
>   *Client:* The child back then had to do it just to survive.
>   *Therapist:* The child back then had to like her father to survive. What about you today?
>   *Client:* Well ... I know that he did a lot of evil things.
>   *Therapist:* Are you saying that perhaps you, the adult, at this moment can feel anger toward your father?

Client: In my head, I guess... but it's very scary to get angry in my heart.
Therapist: What's scary about that?
Client: 'Cause there's so much anger I feel like I might explode.
Therapist: There's so much anger in your heart that you feel you're going to explode. And then, what do you do with that anger? If you keep the anger in your heart, what happens to it?
Client: It turns on me.
Therapist: It turns on you?
Client: I get sick, or hurt myself (long pause).
Therapist: Are you still in the attic with the CHILD?
Client: Yeah, except the ADULT has sat down. She's crying and feeling ashamed.
Therapist: The ADULT has sat down and is crying and feeling ashamed. And how far is the ADULT now from the CHILD?
Client: A couple of feet away.
Therapist: A couple of feet away. What is the CHILD doing right now?
Client: She wants to know what's wrong.
Therapist: She (the CHILD) wants to know what's wrong? And what do you, the ADULT, say to the CHILD? How do you respond to her?
Client: (Crying) "I feel so bad for what I've done to you. I don't deserve to have a relationship with you."
Therapist: And how does the CHILD respond?
Client: "I still want to be with you."
Therapist: She (the CHILD) still wants to be with you. And how do you respond to the CHILD?
Client: I want to say, "I'm sorry, can you forgive me?" but I'm afraid to say that.
Therapist: And what are you afraid of?
Client: That she might forgive me.
Therapist: That she might forgive you? And what scares you about that?

(Therapist employs vertical arrow technique[2] at this point in the imagery.)

Client: That I couldn't lock her in the closet anymore.

Therapist: And if you can't lock her in the closet anymore?

Client: I'd have to accept her and what's happened to her.

Therapist: And if you accept her and what happened to her, then what?

Client: All of a sudden, I don't know if that would be such a bad thing.

Therapist: What would be the worst that could happen if you were to accept her and what happened to her?

Client: I'd have to learn some new behaviors.

Therapist: And what kind of behaviors would you have to give up?

Client: Self-blame and self-hate. I couldn't just automatically blame myself every time something went wrong.

Therapist: Does that scare you, not being able to do that anymore?

Client: Yeah, it does. It would change some of my relationships with people, I think.

Therapist: And how would it change your relationships with people?

Client: On the small level, I would think of them differently.

Therapist: You would think of them differently? And how might you think of them differently?

Client: That if there's any disharmony in the relationship, that maybe it's not me. I might look more realistically at them.

---

2. Rather than challenging the upsetting thoughts directly, the vertical arrow technique involves asking the patient a series of questions (e.g., "If that were true, what would that mean?", "What would happen then?", "What would be so bad about that?") designed to identify the deeper meaning or underlying belief(s) associated with specific upsetting thoughts.

In the imagery that follows, Sarah reveals her fear of seeing others, rather than only herself, as responsible for relationship problems. This fear was associated with an abandonment schema that gave rise to a belief that significant others would leave her if she expected change or equality in the relationship.

Therapist: Does looking at them realistically scare you?
Client: Yeah, because I might lose them.
Therapist: Oh, you might lose them.
Client: But at least I would have myself.
Therapist: But at least you would have yourself?
Client: If I could accept the CHILD and feel more whole, maybe I wouldn't need them the way I do now.
Therapist: So as long as you continue to blame yourself for anything that goes wrong in relationships, then you don't have to fear so much losing the other person. But once you start looking at relationships more realistically—at the other person's role in the relationship—then you recognize that you might lose them, is that it?
Client: Yeah.
Therapist: But you said you would have yourself?
Client: (smiles).
Therapist: What about that made you smile?
Client: It gave me a sense of freedom.
Therapist: What's happening in the attic right now, with you and the CHILD?
Client: I want to ask the CHILD if she'll forgive me.
Therapist: Can you see yourself asking this of the CHILD?
Client: "Will you forgive me?"
Therapist: And how does the CHILD respond?
Client: She just says, "Yes, yes, yes!" and hugs me.
Therapist: The little CHILD comes to you and hugs you. And how are you, the ADULT, responding?
Client: Crying.
Therapist: And how are you feeling?
Client: Less fragmented. More whole.

After eight imagery rescripting sessions, Sarah no longer met criteria for PTSD. Her depression and suicidality significantly diminished, her flashbacks of this abuse episode ceased, and she became more assertive and less dependent in her interactions with family members and friends. Her husband, whose role had been that of caregiver, initially felt threatened as her role of the "sick one" began to change. Following the completion of the eight imagery sessions, several marital sessions were scheduled to help him adjust to Sarah's therapeutic gains. Several months later, Sarah began to experience two new childhood abuse flashbacks, which required two and three imagery rescripting sessions, respectively, to master and eliminate.

12

Case Example 3: Extended IRRT with Higher Order Cognitive/Linguistic Processing

Sharon is a 45-year-old, single, Caucasian woman who was subjected to severe abuse (physical, sexual, and verbal) throughout most of her childhood. Her biological father was an emotionally unstable, abusive alcoholic who married and divorced five women. Sharon's mother was his third wife. He was physically abusive toward Sharon and her mother until he left when Sharon was 3 years old. Sharon continued to have weekend visitations with her father until she turned 18, after which she had no further contact with him. He died when Sharon was in her mid-thirties.

When Sharon was 6, her mother was remarried, to a man who was even more abusive than her biological father had been. Sharon reports that from ages 6 to 16, she was repeatedly subjected to severe physical, sexual, and verbal abuse by her stepfather and her maternal grandmother. Sharon's mother worked as a nurse's aide during the afternoon-evening shift and was not present when the abuse occurred. Sharon also has vivid childhood memories of her mother and sister being subjected to brutal physical and verbal abuse by her stepfather, memories that her sister has recently corroborated. When Sharon was 16, her stepfather left and she never saw him again. He died when Sharon was in her early 40s.

At age 18, Sharon decided to become a nun, which she acknowledges was an attempt to "find refuge," especially from men. At age 23, she left the sisterhood and became involved in a long-term relationship with a man who was physically and verbally abusive toward her. She stayed with him for seven years because she feared she "couldn't live without him." When Sharon finally left him at age 30, she decided to rejoin the sisterhood and has remained a nun since.

Sharon was referred by her female psychiatrist for IRRT because of recurring childhood abuse memories and flashbacks, which had haunted her since early adulthood. In spite of having been in psychotherapy most of her adult life (for over twenty-five years) with many different therapists, Sharon felt she had received very little help with her psychological problems, especially with her chronic PTSD, and was feeling increasingly hopeless and despairing about ever recovering from her painful, debilitating flashbacks. At the time of her referral, Sharon admittedly was struggling daily with whether or not to go on living, and openly stated during her first visit that imagery rescripting was her "last hope."

At the pretreatment evaluation, Sharon clearly met diagnostic criteria for PTSD. She reported suffering for years from daily debilitating physical and sexual childhood abuse flashbacks. In the wake of each intrusive memory, Sharon experienced an overwhelming sense of guilt, shame, self-directed anger, fragmentation, hopelessness, and despair. Sharon's abuse-related cognitions and schemas included viewing herself as powerless, vulnerable, unlovable, inherently bad, defective, alone, rejected, and abandoned. Assessment data gleaned from the Dissociative Experience Scale (DES), Impact of Events Scale–Revised (IES-R), Posttraumatic Symptom Scale (PSS), and the Trauma Symptom Checklist (TSC-40) confirmed that her PTSD symptoms were severe and chronic.

In addition, Sharon reported suffering from severe depression, anxiety, and a pervasive sense of hopelessness, which were corroborated by her high scores on the Beck Depression

Inventory (BDI = 37), Beck Anxiety Inventory (BAI = 44), Beck Hopelessness Scale (BHS = 19), and the Scale for Suicide Ideation (SSI = 25). Sharon's extremely high score on the World Assumptions Scale was a further indication of the pervasiveness of her trauma-related beliefs and her negative views of self and world, as shaped by her childhood traumas and traumagenic schemas.

COURSE OF IMAGERY RESCRIPTING AND REPROCESSING THERAPY

Session 1

Sharon identifies her most upsetting and debilitating flashback to be a physical abuse incident perpetrated by her stepfather when she was 10. She reports experiencing this recurring flashback numerous times weekly over the past eight years. In the following excerpt, the therapist begins the *exposure* phase of imagery.

> *Therapist:* When you're ready, you may close your eyes and visualize the beginning of the abuse scene. When you have a clear image of the abuse, you may begin to describe aloud what you are experiencing, in the present tense, as though it were happening right now.
> *Client:* (long silence; facial grimaces reflect significant distress).
> *Therapist:* Can you verbalize what it is that you're experiencing?
> *Client:* Yes.
> *Therapist:* And what's happening that makes you feel so scared?
> *Client:* It's time for supper and he's not here yet.
> *Therapist:* It's time for supper and he's not here yet?

Client: Right.
Therapist: And where are you?
Client: I'm in the kitchen trying to set the table.

Sharon continues to describe the abuse flashback, in which she nervously anticipates the arrival of her stepfather for dinner. He arrives home late for dinner, drunk, and in a volatile mood. He becomes enraged when he finds that Sharon has not properly set the table. The verbal abuse escalates into physical abuse as he slaps her, pulls her by the hair, and shoves her down the stairs. He then follows her down the stairs and grinds her face into the cement floor with his boot. This image is so vivid for Sharon that she is able to smell the cement. The abuse continues, with more verbal and physical assaults. Finally, when Sharon attempts to call an aunt for help, her stepfather becomes even more enraged. The terror and helplessness become so great that Sharon dissociates in the imagery.

Client: I try to call my aunt, to get help.
Therapist: You try to call your aunt to get help? And what happens when you try to call your aunt?
Client: He comes back.
Therapist: He comes back, and what does he do?
Client: I don't know.
Therapist: What is happening now in the imagery?
Client: I'm frozen.
Therapist: You're frozen?
Client: (long pause).
Therapist: And where are you as you feel frozen?
Client: Sitting on the shelf.
Therapist: You're sitting on a shelf?
Client: In the kitchen.
Therapist: In the kitchen feeling frozen? And what is he doing?
Client: I don't know. He's in the kitchen.

Therapist: He's in the kitchen also? Do you see him there in the kitchen?
Client: Yes.
Therapist: And what do you see him doing?
Client: I can see his mouth going, but I can't hear anything.
Therapist: You see his mouth going, he's continuing to talk to you?
Client: I don't know.
Therapist: You don't even know anymore, you can't hear anything?
Client: Right.
Therapist: Is there anything else that happens in the imagery?
Client: I don't know, I don't think so. I don't know . . . I don't really feel anything.

During the just-completed exposure phase of imagery, Sharon accesses the visual, verbal, sensory, and affective components of her abuse experience, revealing a schema of pervasive powerlessness. As noted by Finkelhor (1990), powerlessness occurs when an individual's will, desires, and sense of efficacy are continually contravened. While even a single traumatic event has the power to inspire helplessness and terror (Morrow and Smith 1995), Sharon's exposure to repeated, ongoing traumas throughout childhood led to the development of a deeply seated, treatment-resistant powerlessness schema, which remains a central theme throughout therapy.

The focus of the imagery session now shifts to rescripting the abuse scene, which involves directly confronting her powerlessness schema. During the rescripting phase that follows, Sharon's powerlessness schema is clarified and challenged through imaginal action and dialogue. The goal of replacing victimization imagery with mastery imagery is met with considerable difficulty.

Therapist: I'd like you now to go back to the very beginning of the flashback and again describe aloud what is happening. This time, however, when we get to a certain place in the flashback, we will change the imagery so that it will have a better outcome for you. I will help you with this. Are you ready to begin?

Sharon nods, indicating she is ready to proceed. She visualizes and verbalizes aloud the same abuse scene. At the height of the abuse, the therapist facilitates the beginning of the rescripting process.

Client: He smashes my face into the cement. I can smell the cement.
Therapist: He smashes your face into the cement and you can smell the cement (brief pause). Can you now visualize yourself today, your ADULT self today, entering the scene at the bottom of the basement stairs? Can you get a picture of that?
Client: (Nods).
Therapist: What do you, the ADULT, do as you enter the scene?
Client: I'm afraid.
Therapist: You're afraid of?
Client: He's too big.
Therapist: Where are you now, you the ADULT?
Client: I'm standing on the last step.
Therapist: You're standing on the last step? Is he aware of your presence?
Client: No.
Therapist: What would you, the ADULT, like to do at this point?
Client: Try to get her away.
Therapist: You'd like to try to get her away? And how would you like to do that?
Client: I'm afraid to touch her because she is really hurt.

Therapist: You're afraid to touch her because she is really hurt? What would you, the ADULT, like to do or say at this point?
Client: I need to get rid of him. I don't know how to make him leave.
Therapist: You need to get rid of him, but you don't know how? So what would you like to do to him to make him leave?
Client: I just want to move her [the CHILD]. I don't care about him.
Therapist: You want to just move her, but you said you need to get rid of him first, to get him out of the way? Is that what you said?
Client: But there's no way to do that. He's just there.
Therapist: He's just there? There's no way you feel you can get him out of the way?
Client: I have to get her out of there (voice beginning to sound desperate). This is too much!

At this point, Sharon holds both hands to her head and seems to be saying to the therapist that the pain is more than she can handle. Even though Sharon is obviously experiencing a great deal of emotional pain at this moment, it is crucial that she stay with the pain and continue to confront her powerlessness schema while struggling to develop more adaptive coping strategies. Circumventing the trauma-related pain at this point (e.g., through dissociating or stopping the imagery) would be succumbing to her powerlessness schema and would further reinforce her sense of helplessness and victimization.

Therapist: So how do you get her [the CHILD] out of there?
Client: (Long silence).
Therapist: So how do you, the ADULT, get him away from her so that you can get her [the CHILD] out of there?
Client: (10 seconds) I don't know.

> *Therapist:* What would you like to do to him at this point? If you could, what would you like to do?
> *Client:* I don't know.
> *Therapist:* You don't know?
> *Client:* I'm so afraid.
> *Therapist:* You're so afraid of him? You, the ADULT, are so afraid of him?
> *Client:* Yes.

Sharon's powerlessness schema is so strong that it prevents her from visualizing herself as an adult today confronting and removing her stepfather from the abuse scene. In such instances, it is sometimes helpful to ask the patient if an object or weapon might be useful. Sharon, however, declines to even attempt this intervention because of her fear that "he would do me in if I didn't accomplish it the first time." As a last resort, the therapist invites the ADULT to bring a support person into the imagery to help out.

> *Therapist:* What about bringing a police officer into the imagery?
> *Client:* I don't think it would do any good.
> *Therapist:* You don't think it would do any good to have several armed policemen there?
> *Client:* I don't know. It just feels so helpless.
> *Therapist:* Is that something you would be willing to try?
> *Client:* (deep sigh) Sure.

Sharon reluctantly agrees to conduct a "behavioral experiment" in the imagery. It is crucial that Sharon not end the first rescripted imagery session before experiencing some increased sense of empowerment vis-à-vis the perpetrator, even if it means bringing in other people to do the work for her.

> *Therapist:* Would you want to bring in one or several police officers?

Client: It would take more than one.
Therapist: How many would you want to bring in?
Client: Four or five.
Therapist: Okay. Can you now visualize four or five police officers there?
Client: Yes.
Therapist: And where are these police officers in relation to your stepfather?
Client: They're trying to restrain him.
Therapist: They're trying to restrain him. And how is he responding?
Client: He's very angry.... He keeps swearing at them and telling them that it's none of their business.
Therapist: And how do the police officers respond?
Client: They put handcuffs on him and keep trying to make him be quiet.... They're now trying to escort him out of the building.
Therapist: They're trying to escort him out of the building? And how is he responding?
Client: He's quite abusive, verbally.
Therapist: What is he saying?
Client: He keeps calling them names and telling them that it's none of their business, that this is a family matter.

Sharon then visualizes the officers putting handcuffs on her stepfather and physically removing him from the home. Although the stepfather continues to put up considerable resistance, the five policemen are eventually able to subdue him and take him off to jail. Sharon also visualizes two of the officers talking to her, the ADULT, in a sympathetic, nurturing manner, expressing how sorry they are that this happened, that "this should not happen to anybody." Sharon seems puzzled and can't understand why they feel sorry for her (a direct contradiction to her unlovable schema). The therapist attempts to understand her reaction by inquiring about her related cognitions.

Therapist: When they say that this shouldn't happen to anybody, what thoughts go through your mind?
Client: I keep feeling this wave of sadness. I don't want to feel that, it feels too much!
Therapist: You keep feeling this wave of sadness that feels just overwhelming, overbearing?
Client: Yes.
Therapist: What's happening now in the imagery?
Client: Nothing.
Therapist: What's happening with your stepfather and the policemen outside?
Client: They took him away to jail.
Therapist: They take him to jail. And what's happening now with you, the ADULT, and the CHILD in the house?
Client: We're just sitting there.

Sharon appears to have completed the mastery imagery phase of rescripting. The therapist facilitates the transition to the ADULT–CHILD phase of imagery, in which she visualizes her ADULT responding to her CHILD. Not surprisingly, Sharon has much difficulty with this phase of imagery.

Therapist: You, the ADULT, and the CHILD are just sitting there? And what would you, the ADULT, like to do or say to the CHILD?
Client: (5 seconds) "I'm so sorry."
Therapist: And how does the CHILD respond?
Client: She just looks.
Therapist: And what do you, the ADULT, see in the CHILD's face, in her eyes?
Client: It's just empty.... She's just sitting there staring.

During the ADULT–CHILD imagery, Sharon's ADULT and CHILD are unable to form an emotional connection. The CHILD is unresponsive to the ADULT's nurturing efforts, and the CHILD has an empty, autistic-like gaze in her eyes, all of which suggests that self-abuse is a serious problem for Sharon. Individuals subjected to severe abuse as children frequently report engaging in self-abusive behavior as adults in an attempt to hurt, punish, or even destroy the "child" within, whom they blame for the abuse and whom they regard as inherently bad, evil, and unlovable.[1] It is as though the CHILD in the imagery "knows" this, feels threatened by the ADULT, and thus tries to self-protect by not allowing the ADULT to get close.

Throughout the remainder of the imagery session, Sharon continues to visualize the CHILD as totally unresponsive, even as the ADULT cleans up the CHILD, holds and rocks her, and puts her to bed. During post-imagery session processing, Sharon reports feeling relieved at "seeing" her stepfather being taken away by the police, but also frustrated with not being able to "reach" the CHILD during the imagery session. For homework, Sharon is given an audiotape of the entire imagery session, which she is instructed to listen to daily.

Session 2

The imaginal exposure to the abuse flashback in this session closely parallels that of the previous session. During the mastery imagery phase of rescripting, Sharon again needs the assistance of five policemen to "rescue" the CHILD from

---

1. According to introject theory, self-abusive individuals have developed an abusive "perpetrator introject." Abuse victims often continue to treat themselves as they were treated by their perpetrators. This may be evidenced during ADULT-CHILD imagery when the ADULT appears to take on the role of the perpetrator (e.g., becoming impatient, angry, or abusive toward the CHILD) and the CHILD takes on the role of the victimized child.

the abuse scene. This time, however, Sharon's ADULT seems less terrified of her stepfather, as she visualizes him being quiet and subdued while handcuffed and taken away by the policemen, suggesting the beginning of a shift in her powerlessness schema. Throughout the ADULT–CHILD imagery, the CHILD is again totally unresponsive to the ADULT and continues to exhibit autistic-like behaviors throughout (e.g., tapping, rocking), despite numerous attempts by the ADULT to reach out and nurture the CHILD.

During the post-imagery debriefing, Sharon complains how painful the imagery was for her, that she felt more physical and emotional pain this time. She admits starting to feel some anger at her stepfather, which terrifies her, especially since she has never before allowed herself to feel any anger toward him. A discussion ensues exploring Sharon's beliefs and religious assumptions regarding anger. Her belief that any expression of anger is "un-Christlike" is identified and challenged. Through a Socratic dialogue facilitated by the therapist, Sharon begins to see that anger is a normal human emotion, that even Jesus displayed anger at times, and that being a good Christian does *not* mean never allowing oneself to get angry. When a patient holds maladaptive views of anger that appear linked to his/her religious beliefs, it is crucial that the patient's views of anger be examined and challenged from within the patient's (not the therapist's) religious frame of reference.

Session 3

Sharon appears to have benefited from the discussion about anger in the previous session, as she openly expresses anger toward her stepfather for the first time. At one point in the exposure phase of imagery, she spontaneously blurts out, "I hate him so much!" During the mastery imagery phase, her posture also changes dramatically.

> *Therapist:* If you could, what would you like to do at this point, you the ADULT?
> *Client:* Make him leave.
> *Therapist:* And how would you like to make him leave?
> *Client:* Push him through the wall.
> *Therapist:* Push him through the wall? Physically push him through the wall?
> *Client:* Yes, to make him stop.
> *Therapist:* Can you get a picture of you, the ADULT, doing just that, pushing him through the wall?
> *Client:* Yes.

The idea of pushing her stepfather through the wall comes from Sharon, *not* from the therapist. The therapist merely asks Sharon if she can visualize herself enacting the coping strategy that she herself has verbalized.

> *Therapist:* What happens when you push him through the wall?
> *Client:* He just goes through the wall.

No longer needing the assistance of five armed policemen, Sharon is now able to remove the perpetrator from the abuse scene herself. This marks an important shift in her powerlessness schema, as she no longer perceives herself as a helpless victim frozen in a state of powerlessness. In the ADULT–CHILD phase of imagery that follows, however, Sharon continues to have difficulty establishing an emotional connection with the CHILD, who remains "in hiding" under the steps.

> *Therapist:* What would you like to do with the little girl?
> *Client:* Try to get her to come out.
> *Therapist:* And how would you like to try to do that?
> *Client:* Convince her that he can't hurt her right now.
> *Therapist:* Can you see yourself doing that?
> *Client:* I keep trying to take her hand, but she won't take my hand.

Therapist: How does she respond?
Client: She doesn't, she just sits there rocking back and forth.
Therapist: You ask her what she wants you to do and she doesn't respond? So you're not sure if she wants you to stay or to leave. Is that right?
Client: Right.
Therapist: Could you ask her directly if she wants you to stay or leave?
Client: "Do you want me to stay or go away?"
Therapist: And how does she respond?
Client: She just put out her hand.
Therapist: She puts out her hand toward you? And how do you respond?
Client: I try to take her hand, but she takes it away.

Reaching out her hand toward the ADULT denotes the first sign of any kind that the CHILD may want to connect with the ADULT. Yet, there is still much ambivalence and fear that the CHILD feels vis-à-vis the ADULT, as reflected in her pulling her hand back the moment the ADULT tries to take it. The CHILD does eventually go with the ADULT upstairs to the bathroom to get cleaned up, but remains suspicious and emotionally distant from the ADULT, which continues to frustrate and upset Sharon.

Sessions 4 Through 7

During the next four sessions, Sharon is able to experience the imaginal exposure phase of the flashback with progressively less emotionality, while continuing to visualize herself as an adult confronting and removing the perpetrator from the abuse scene with increased ease in the mastery/rescripting phase. Yet Sharon's frustration with the ADULT–CHILD phase of imagery continues to build as the CHILD remains unresponsive. After seven sessions of imaginal exposure and rescripting, Sharon has gained sufficient mastery over the abuse imagery of the flashback and seems ready to proceed to the ADULT–CHILD only phase of imagery.

Sessions 8 and 9

During these ADULT–CHILD imagery sessions, Sharon's frustration and impatience with the CHILD continue to increase. It seems that no matter what the ADULT does, or how the ADULT attempts to reach out to the CHILD, the CHILD remains mute and unresponsive, and continues to sit on the floor rocking and tapping with the same empty, autistic-like gaze in her eyes. Sharon's lifelong unlovable/self-hatred schema, it seems, lies at the core of her difficulties with self-nurturance, which are so vividly and poignantly portrayed in the ADULT–CHILD imagery.

Session 10

At the beginning of the session, Sharon's homework record indicates zero SUDs ratings (i.e., a complete absence of affect) on many of the days while listening to the audiotape of the previous ADULT–CHILD imagery session. Further questioning reveals that the zero SUDs scores are a result of Sharon's dissociating in the imagery because "it is too painful to stay with the feelings." This is followed by a brief discussion about the nature and history of her abuse-related pain, how Sharon has attempted unsuccessfully to cope with that pain throughout her life, how she feels hopelessly stuck in her pain, and how the only way for her to get beyond the pain is to work through it in a meaningful way. Sharon also complains about the loud, critical voices in her head (an auditory activation of her hostile introjects) that make it difficult for her to listen to the imagery tapes between sessions.

Client: I have trouble controlling all the noise in my head, the loud voices.
Therapist: And what are the loud voices saying?
Client: They are very, very critical. . . . It has to do with that I talk too much, that I reveal too many things and then I don't feel safe, the mechanisms that I use to protect myself aren't there.
Therapist: And whose voices or voice is telling you that stuff?
Client: My stepfather and my grandmother. I can see their faces, I can hear their voices, like they're sitting there at the table next to me saying that no one outside the family is entitled to this information.
Therapist: So it's your stepfather's and your grandmother's voices?
Client: And sometimes it feels like my own. I really feel little and really scared, like "now you did it again and you're going to pay for this."
Therapist: You feel like you've betrayed your stepfather and grandmother and now you will pay for this? And how do you pay for this?
Client: It's what I do to myself sometimes, self-abuse and not taking very good care of myself.

To date, Sharon has not been willing to share the specifics of her self-abuse. She reports, however, feeling a sense of temporary relief from her emotional pain when she self-abuses, as the critical voices become quieter for awhile, all of which highly reinforces and strengthens her unlovable/worthlessness schema.

In the ADULT–CHILD imagery that follows, Sharon initially reports difficulty "seeing" the CHILD, who is darting in and out of a dark room and closet (the room that she and her sister shared while Sharon was in the seventh grade). When the ADULT enters the imagery scene, the CHILD stops darting and is sitting in the back of the closet, leaning against the wall and feeling nervous. The ADULT is on the opposite side of the room from the CHILD. When asked what she, the ADULT, would like to do or say to the CHILD, the ADULT's response is "convince her [the CHILD] to come out of the closet and take her to a safe place." The CHILD responds to the ADULT's invitation with skepticism and mistrust.

> *Client:* "It's okay for you to come with me. You have to get out."
> *Therapist:* And how does little Sharon respond?
> *Client:* She's not sure if she can trust it.
> *Therapist:* What is she afraid of?
> *Client:* It just feels safer in the closet, three walls and a door, she knows exactly what's in there.
> *Therapist:* And how do you, the ADULT, respond to her fears of coming out and going to a safe place?
> *Client:* I'm trying to figure out the best way that I can handle this.
> *Therapist:* So you, the ADULT, hear her concerns and her fears of coming out. You'd like to get her to a safe place, get her out of there, but are not sure of what the best way to handle it is? And you feel that there might be some legitimacy to her concerns?
> *Client:* Yes.

It is crucial that the therapist *not* put words in the patient's mouth, but merely reflect back what the patient has already said or what the therapist senses the patient may be trying to say.

> *Therapist:* Can you say that to her directly?
> *Client:* "I understand how it feels."
> *Therapist:* And?
> *Client:* I don't know.
> *Therapist:* And what's the rest of what you want to say to her?

> *Client:* We need to get out, but I don't know where to go.
> *Therapist:* "I understand how you feel. I'd like to take you out to safety somewhere, but I'm not sure where. Yet I understand why you are afraid to do that, why you are afraid to come out." Is that what you're saying to her?
> *Client:* Yes.
> *Therapist:* So you really understand her fears?
> *Client:* Yes.

In general, when the ADULT is able to express genuine empathy to the CHILD during ADULT–CHILD imagery, the CHILD becomes more responsive to, and accepting of, the ADULT.

> *Therapist:* And how does little Sharon respond to you when you let her know that you understand her fears, that you would like to take her to safety, but that you very well understand that she is afraid to come out? How does little Sharon respond?
> *Client:* She had been leaning against the wall and pushing with her feet, but now she's leaning forward like she's trying to listen.
> *Therapist:* Now she's leaning forward toward you more?
> *Client:* Yes.
> *Therapist:* Like she's trying to listen?
> *Client:* She has her hands on her lap and she's leaning forward looking down.

This marks the first time during any of the ADULT–CHILD imagery sessions that the CHILD has responded favorably to any of the ADULT's overtures. It appears that the ADULT has, for the first time, been able to empathize directly with the CHILD's fears. However, the ADULT's empathy for the CHILD is short-lived and is quickly replaced by the ADULT's fears of not being safe.

Client: "I'm really worried, we have to get out of here. We can't take a long time to think about this. We just have to get out of here" (agitation and sense of panic reflected in voice).
Therapist: I'm worried that if we don't?
Client: Something is going to happen.
Therapist: Something is going to happen if we don't get out?
Client: We have to get out soon.
Therapist: How does little Sharon respond?
Client: She keeps tapping her fingers, but she doesn't look up. She keeps looking down and rocking and tapping her fingers. I keep trying to tell her we can't wait anymore, we have to go.
Therapist: And how does she respond?
Client: She seems really nervous again. She's afraid to move.

The connection that was beginning to develop between the CHILD and the ADULT quickly disappears, as the ADULT's tone becomes increasingly agitated and demanding. The therapist now faces the challenge of facilitating a reconnection between the ADULT and CHILD while remaining Socratic and nondirective.

Therapist: A few minutes ago when you had reflected back to the CHILD that you understood her concerns and her fears, she had relaxed more then?
Client: Yes, it seems like it.
Therapist: And now when you tell her very emphatically, "We must get out of here, we have to go now," like there's no tomorrow; when you say that to her with that sense of desperation in your voice, she gets more nervous?
Client: Yes.

Therapist: Why do you think she gets more nervous when you talk to her that way?

Client: It's too scary out there, she knows what's in the closet. She's stuck. I don't want to leave her. We have to get out.

Therapist: And how is she responding?

Client: She's rocking and tapping her fingers.

Therapist: Are you noticing that she responds to you differently depending on how calm or upset you are?

Client: Yes, I think so.

Therapist: Earlier it seemed like you were calmer, you were showing understanding and empathy toward her. And when you conveyed that to her she not only seemed calmer but she began to lean forward toward you, like she wanted to hear more. Then your voice shifted and you began to feel afraid, almost a sense of desperation. Then you said to her, "We have to get out of here!" And then she started to respond differently, the tapping, the rocking, is that right? Am I hearing that right?

Client: Yes.

Therapist: So might there be something in the way that you express yourself to her, in your demeanor that she responds to?

Client: I think so.

Therapist: And how would you put that into words?

Client: I'm remembering how painful it is. Makes me want to run, like there's no tomorrow.

Therapist: And when you, the ADULT, feel that and convey that to little Sharon, how does she respond?

Client: She gets stiff as a board. There's no way to think. There's too much stimulation. There's no way to take it in, she stays stiff. Too much, she can't listen anymore.

Therapist: But earlier when you were calmer, then she was calmer, then she could take in what you had to say?

Client: Yeah.

The goal at this point in the imagery is for the ADULT to calm herself so that she can approach the CHILD in a way that the CHILD can trust, accept, and feel safe responding to. In the previous nine sessions, however, the ADULT has expressed agitation, frustration, and fear during the ADULT–CHILD imagery, responding much more like a frightened child than a competent, nurturing adult. The challenge for the therapist is to remain patient and nondirective while continuing with the Socratic imagery. Sharon has the ability to self-calm and self-nurture, which she demonstrated briefly a few minutes earlier when her ADULT was feeling calmer vis-à-vis the CHILD. The therapist's task now is to help Sharon reconnect with that part of herself.

Therapist: How did you get yourself to be calmer earlier, when you were feeling calmer inside and that was reflected in how you expressed yourself? How did you get yourself to be calmer inside then?
Client: I saw the light in my head, and when I would take a breath I could move the light down.
Therapist: And that helped you get calmer inside?
Client: Yes.
Therapist: Is that something that you could do now as a way of calming yourself again?
Client: Yes.
Therapist: You see the light in your head, and then what?

Although the therapist had no previous knowledge of the light image and the breathing Sharon mentions, and is unclear where she is going with this, Sharon's ADULT seems to know. It is therefore crucial that the therapist not interfere or attempt to guide. By remaining non-directive, the therapist reinforces Sharon's efforts to help herself as she takes the lead in tapping into and utilizing her own psychological resources.

Client: I take a deep breath and try to move the light down.
Therapist: Are you doing that now?
Client: Yes.
Therapist: And how is that affecting your level of calmness or upsetness?
Client: My stomach doesn't hurt.
Therapist: Are you feeling calmer again?
Client: Yes.
Therapist: Does little Sharon see that you're becoming calmer again?
Client: She must because she's not rocking anymore.
Therapist: So once again as you, the ADULT, become calmer inside, the CHILD looks like she is becoming calmer, less anxious, less fearful? Is that what's happening?
Client: Yes.
Therapist: What would you, the ADULT, like to do or say to the CHILD at this point, now that you've returned to your calmer state?
Client: "It's okay to come out" (voice calm and reassuring).
Therapist: It's okay to come out?
Client: "I'll stay right here at the door and you can sit on my lap."
Therapist: And how does little Sharon respond?
Client: She's sitting on my lap now (appears surprised).
Therapist: As she's now sitting on your lap, how are you, the ADULT, responding?
Client: I'm sitting with my hands on my knees and she puts my hands together. She just holds them together with hers.
Therapist: And how are you, the ADULT, responding?
Client: I can't believe this!
Therapist: You can't believe this?
Client: I have to stay calm.
Therapist: You're beginning to realize that you need to stay calm if you're going to be able to help her. Is that what you're saying?

EXTENDED IRRT WITH HIGHER ORDER PROCESSING

> *Client:* That's what it feels like.
> *Therapist:* That's what it feels like. Which part of this can't you believe?
> *Client:* That she's sitting here.
> *Therapist:* That she's sitting here on your lap?
> *Client:* And that we are that close.

Sharon now appears to have entered a calm and relaxed state. Her voice is calm and soothing, her breathing is slow and deep, and the muscles throughout her body appear relaxed.

> *Therapist:* Are you saying that you were not aware, when you get upset, how much that upsets and scares her [the CHILD]? You weren't aware of that connection before?
> *Client:* Right.
> *Therapist:* And how when you're calm, then she's not only able to be calmer but she's calm enough to be able to come to you and be close with you. Is that what you're saying and seeing?
> *Client:* Right.
> *Therapist:* What's happening now in the imagery?

The therapist attempts to facilitate a shift from secondary cognitive processing back to primary cognitive processing. However, Sharon has a need for further secondary cognitive processing, which the therapist appropriately goes along with.

> *Client:* It feels so comfortable (tears well up in Sharon's eyes).
> *Therapist:* It feels so comfortable. You look like you're crying or about ready to cry. What's that about?
> *Client:* It's very comforting.
> *Therapist:* It's so comforting it makes you want to cry? Tears of joy almost?
> *Client:* Yes.
> *Therapist:* And what is so comforting about this?

Client: Just to be that close.

Therapist: Just to be that close. You've been working for a long time at getting closer to that little girl, haven't you?

Client: Yes.

Therapist: You've been trying so hard and have at times felt quite upset and desperate about not being able to get closer to that little girl. She has never come to you like this before.

Client: Right.

Therapist: And now you find today that all you need to do is to calm yourself, you the ADULT, and then she comes to you like this?

Client: Right.

The therapist again facilitates a shift back to primary cognitive processing, for which Sharon now seems ready.

Therapist: What's happening now in the imagery?

Client: She keeps running her hands over the top of my hands.

Therapist: And how does that feel?

Client: I'm just so surprised . . .

Therapist: Is there anything that you, the ADULT, would like to say to the CHILD as she is sitting on your lap with her hands in your hands?

Client: Thank you.

Therapist: Thank you, you say to her?

Client: (crying, nods).

Therapist: And how does little Sharon respond?

Client: She puts her head back against my face, on the side of my neck.

Therapist: And how does that feel?

Client: It doesn't feel so lonely.

Therapist: It doesn't feel so lonely?

Client: And very soft . . . .

Sharon then discovers that she no longer feels rushed to get out of the house, the house that minutes before felt so ominous and foreboding. Sharon also observes that the CHILD's face no longer looks so worried and distressed. The imagery eventually winds down with the CHILD and ADULT sitting together in the light, the CHILD still sitting comfortably on the ADULT's lap, the ADULT's arms wrapped around her, and the two rocking together feeling close and calm.

In the post-imagery processing and debriefing, the therapist notes Sharon's dramatically changed mood and then asks Sharon what she has learned from the session.

Therapist: Well, you're smiling.
Client: I wish you could have been there!
Therapist: In a sense I was there. (pause) You really had this look of surprise and shock on your face when she [the CHILD] first came over to you.
Client: I never thought I'd see the day.
Therapist: Now what have you learned from this today? What is the most important thing that you've learned from this imagery session today?
Client: It was being able to see the light. And as I took each breath, having the light move down and just feeling myself get so much more calm, and not feeling so frantic inside, like something terrible is always going to happen.
Therapist: And you have the ability to calm yourself down like this. Did you know that you had that ability before?
Client: I did a long time ago, but it's just...
Therapist: It's just what?
Client: I feel like I've been revved-up for so long that I've forgotten things that are soothing.
Therapist: You've forgotten how to self-soothe, self-calm, and self-nurture, haven't you? I guess what you've experienced today is that you still have the power within

you to do that. Look at yourself now! And when you're able to calm yourself like this, look at what happens! You feel a connection with that little girl that you never felt before. This is the very first time, isn't it?
Client: It's the very first time.

Sharon takes the audiotape of the imagery session home and listens to it daily for the purpose of reinforcing the self-nurturing, self-calming images and feelings she has experienced during the session. Sharon is also asked to practice using the light imagery together with the deep breathing between sessions as a means of calming herself, especially when feeling upset.

The above ADULT–CHILD imagery session marks a significant breakthrough in Sharon's therapy. Following this session, Sharon reports a virtual cessation of this particular flashback. Not only has Sharon gained mastery over the specific recurring abuse flashback involving her stepfather, she has also begun to make significant inroads in actively challenging her lifelong unlovable schema. She does, however, report the continued presence of other recurring flashbacks from childhood traumas that involve stepfather- and grandmother-perpetrated sexual abuse. Through additional imagery rescripting sessions, Sharon is able to successfully confront and emotionally process each additional flashback. Generally, three to five imagery rescripting sessions are needed for Sharon to successfully confront and emotionally process each additional recurring flashback she experiences. Although the pain associated with the activation of Sharon's flashbacks is often quite intense, and she at times resorts to dissociating in the imagery as a means of numbing herself to the pain, Sharon nonetheless shows a great deal of stamina, courage, and perseverance in staying with and processing the painful traumatic imagery in her struggle to gain mastery over her recurring flashbacks and abuse memories.

HIGHER ORDER COGNITIVE/LINGUISTIC PROCESSING

In spite of the significant progress Sharon has made with her flashbacks, she still does not feel a sense of complete mastery over them and remains frightened of the flashbacks and flashback fragments she continues to experience from time to time. In an effort to more fully process her abuse experiences and memories, a greater degree of integration of the emotional and linguistic elements of the abuse is sought. Sharon is asked to transform the visual, verbal, auditory, and kinesthetic sensations of her recurring traumatic memories into written language as part of her homework assignments. These assignments include writing a narrative of her traumatic abuse experiences and her reactions to each abuse memory. In addition, Sharon agrees to (1) type out transcripts from the audiotapes of each imagery rescripting session (including the exposure, mastery, and ADULT–CHILD phases of imagery), (2) insert her own commentary parenthetically into the transcripts as she types them, and (3) record her reactions to the transcript writing process itself. While Sharon was understandably somewhat fearful of immersing herself in such an assignment, she complied nonetheless and was very pleased with the results. She reported that the transcript-writing work greatly enhanced her sense of mastery over the flashbacks and seemed to foster a higher level of emotional-linguistic processing of her traumatic memories. The following is an excerpt from Sharon's description of what the imagery rescripting transcript writing was like for her:

> The very first transcript that I did, I felt pretty detached. But as I began to write out the next transcript, I began to experience a physiological response I did not like. There was tremendous fear and anxiety that I would be overcome by the flashbacks because I wasn't sure I was strong enough to handle them.

Little by little, however, I learned that in writing the transcript that is in front of me, I feel that I have some control over how fast the images are coming. It's like watching a movie and being able to control the speed of each frame of the film. I have time to pause, let myself feel, and still recover on my own. Being able to pull out of a dissociative state can take place because I can look around the room and know that this house, this room is nothing like the room or house in which the abuse took place.

The transcripts provide a written tool, but they also enable me to hear in my head what actually takes place between me and my doctor. Because he repeats everything I say, it not only enables me to realize that I am heard, but it also validates my truth, my experience. While I am recalling the event of the flashback, I can hear my doctor's voice in my head. Voice contact helps me recall the event, but also keeps me in touch with the here and now.

In the weeks and months that follow, the cognitive therapy sessions with Sharon involve both imagery and nonimagery work. While gaining mastery over all recurring flashbacks remains a central goal of therapy, a concomitant goal is for Sharon to transfer the cognitive/behavioral coping strategies she develops during the imagery rescripting sessions to everyday life situations. In particular, the self-calming and self-soothing imagery she creates, in conjunction with the light imagery and the deep breathing, becomes a potent coping strategy to use in stressful and upsetting situations. Much practice and additional therapeutic work are needed, however, before Sharon is able to successfully apply these self-calming coping strategies to external, day-to-day situations.

In spite of the progress Sharon is making with her flashbacks, she continues to blame herself for her abuse and victimization and cannot imagine herself ever being anything but damaged and ruined from the abuse. The following excerpts from her writings reflect the core schemas of defectiveness, unlovability, and mistrust that continue to have a grip on her view of self:

What I have thought and continue to think is that he ruined me for life and no matter what I do or how hard I work, that fact will never change.... My belief about myself is that deep down to the core, I am this horrible wretch of a person....

I blame myself for my abuse. In the beginning when I was much younger, it was naturally my fault because I could never seem to be the kind of person my parents wanted or needed. It was my fault that my parents divorced. It was my fault that my mother's second marriage didn't work and that I seemed to make them so angry. When everything began with my stepfather, he said I egged him on, so what I got I deserved. As time went on, and to this day, my thoughts are that if I wasn't who I was, life would be so different for everyone who knows me and who has anything to do with me....

Trusting other people is very hard. My experience has been that trust is very difficult, i.e., either I don't trust at all or I trust the wrong people for all the wrong reasons....

Most of the time I feel like a total failure in relationships and that I don't have a clue how to be in or maintain one at all. I don't trust myself. I have encounters with people and come away feeling horribly inadequate....

You have to work hard just to survive and you should not expect to be happy. Happiness and joy come to other people, not me.

In spite of the therapist's attempts to confront, challenge, and modify Sharon's traumagenic schemas, it seems that such efforts are to no avail. At the moment, Sharon seems stuck in her victimization and self-hatred.

As the therapist begins to explore more aggressively with Sharon possible causes of her inability to move forward, Sharon confesses a secret, to which she has only made vague allusions in previous sessions. Unbeknownst to the therapist, as well as to all of Sharon's former therapists, is her twenty-nine-year history of self-abuse, which began at age 16, when her stepfather left home. It appears that when the stepfather-perpetrated abuse ceased, the self-abuse began. The self-abuse involves Sharon inserting either a coat hanger or a knitting needle vaginally until she hurts and bleeds. According to Sharon, she can tolerate self-induced physical pain much better than emotional pain, which she finds unbearable. During periods of intense emotional distress, Sharon "hears" loud, angry voices in her head telling her how bad, despicable, and worthless she is. At such times, when Sharon feels emotionally overwhelmed and defeated by the voices, she engages in physical and sexual self-abuse in order to "silence the voices and escape the pain." Sharon also feels she deserves to be punished in this way because she is such a "bad" person.

The voices that Sharon hears in her head are best conceptualized as an auditory activation of her own hostile introjects and should not be confused with voices a schizophrenic might hear. Sharon is fully aware that these voices are a form of negative self-talk inside her own head. Although she may become very upset by the voices and often has difficulty quieting them, Sharon knows that these voices have no external reality (i.e., they do not exist outside of her own head).

Sharon reports she has been self-abusing in this way on a regular basis for twenty-nine years, ranging from several times a week to several times daily. While this self-abuse is no doubt a form of self-inflicted punishment that serves to reinforce and perpetuate her bad/unlovable schema, engaging in these self-injurious behaviors also appears to be Sharon's primitive attempt to self-calm and self-soothe during times of emotional distress and suffering. Indeed, Sharon does report feeling better immediately after she self-abuses; that is, the voices become silent and she feels calmer, for a while.

At this point in treatment, the focus is entirely on the self-abuse. Sharon is told she must stop her primitive, self-injurious behaviors totally and completely before any further progress in therapy can be made. Directly confronting and modifying her bad/unlovable schema, as well as finding healthier, more adaptive ways to self-calm and self-soothe when she is upset become vital treatment goals for Sharon. To achieve this goal, Sharon must first come to understand that her self-abusive behaviors are unacceptable, primitive, addictive-like behaviors that need to be stopped, and that nobody—herself included—deserves such treatment. This is initially quite difficult for Sharon to accept, as her self-abuse is so intertwined with her unlovable schema. To stop the self-abuse because she does not deserve such treatment is a direct affront and challenge to her core schematic belief: "I am inherently unlovable and deserve to be punished." Nonetheless, Sharon agrees to contract with the therapist to call him, day or night, before injuring herself in any way.

Not surprisingly, Sharon has some initial difficulty honoring the contract. The therapist responds by confronting her firmly, but in a caring manner, repeating that the self-abusive behavior is not acceptable, and that she must find other ways to cope with her emotional pain when the hostile voices are activated. Numerous imagery interventions are used to assist Sharon with this, including visualizing her therapist confronting and overwhelming the hostile voices, listening to audiotapes of her therapist using humor to disempower the voices (e.g., mimicking the voices using a high-pitched, squeaky voice—an intervention that Sharon finds outrageously funny and that brings her to laughter every time she listens to the audiotape).

Needless to say, the therapeutic relationship is most critical when working with patients like Sharon, and unquestionably becomes the primary vehicle through which significant cognitive/schema/introject change occurs. A primary therapeutic task for Sharon thus is to internalize the secure base of the therapy sessions by developing a positive therapist introject (i.e., an internal visual/auditory cognitive representation of the therapist) to replace her hostile introjects. To accomplish this, Sharon must feel trustful of and connected with her therapist, so that she can internalize the therapist's calming/reassuring voice and mentally activate it as a means of self-calming and self-soothing during times of emotional distress, especially when she feels overpowered by the negative, hostile voices within.

SUMMARY

In the weeks and months that follow, Sharon is able to make slow but substantial progress at developing a positive therapist introject. Gradually, she develops a greatly enhanced ability to self-calm and self-soothe when feeling upset. Sharon's increased repertoire of cognitive tools has helped her to develop stronger emotional shock absorbers, so that she can better absorb the daily knocks of life without being thrown into a major crisis whenever she goes over a bump in the road.

As Sharon enters the latter phase of treatment, her therapy becomes more here-and-now focused, with a much greater emphasis on implementing a variety of cognitive-behavioral coping strategies on her own between sessions. Yet Sharon continues to report that it is only when she can hear the supportive voice of her therapist from within (as well as that of her psychiatrist and spiritual leader) that she is able to successfully apply on her own any of the cognitive-behavioral coping strategies she has learned (e.g., self-calming imagery interventions involving the light and deep breathing, visualizing her therapist confront the voices, asserting herself in stressful work situations, coping with additional abuse flashbacks that emerge). According to introject theory, one would expect that as Sharon continues in her recovery, she will have internalized her therapist's voice to such a degree that she will no longer be able to distinguish it from her own voice, that in effect her therapist's voice becomes her own voice.

Sharon's final hurdle in her recovery at present is perhaps her biggest challenge to date: finding meaning in her abuse and recognizing the strength she has gained from her recovery work. The therapist is now challenging Sharon more aggressively in this endeavor, contending that the time has now come for her to take this final step. A concern that Sharon keeps articulating is her fear that her therapist will abandon her if and when she takes this step. Although the therapist has continually attempted to reassure Sharon that the therapy will not end until she (Sharon) decides it is time, Sharon's abandonment schema continues to interfere with her efforts to find meaning to her abuse. The following are excerpts from her most recent homework assignment relating to this:

> On my first day of imagery rescripting, I remember telling my therapist that he was "my last hope." I had been through the wringer in terms of therapies [over 25 years of therapy] and was feeling that I had no hope for any future. For so long I had been feeling desperate to find a purpose to my suffering and a sense of direction, but I kept coming up with no good reason to prolong my life any further.
>
> Since working with Dr. S., I have made significant progress in being able to control the flashbacks instead of them controlling me. Though I have been able to have some wonderful positive experiences recently, I have felt emotionally detached from them, as if it wasn't really me who was there, but someone else in my place. This someone I call my "ambassador." The ambassador is very capable and organized, likable and very funny.
>
> When the ambassador isn't activated, I feel terribly threatened by too much praise. It is hard to allow myself the experience of much-needed feedback because of my fear that I will never be able to maintain this and then people will see me for who I really am and will abandon me. I believe this fear has kept me from being able to integrate these positive parts in a meaningful way.
>
> When I was first asked to read Viktor Frankl's *Man's Search for Meaning*, I felt some resistance inside because I couldn't see how surviving concentration camps could speak to my own life experience. As I began reading Frankl's account

of the cruelty, torture, humiliation, and what had to be done just to survive one more day, memories of my own abuse began surfacing. Vivid, almost paralyzing memories of what my own perpetrators inflicted helped me to see that the treatment I received had had similar effects. Being treated less than human, forced to do things, to endure things that little by little ate away at my self-esteem until there was very little left of a viable human being.

Frankl speaks of being able to endure such terrible things by calling up an image of his wife. Being able to see her, in his mind saying things to her and having her answer was a way for him to cope with the unthinkable. In my own experience (prior to imagery rescripting), I could not call up an image of such a person. Even turning to God and the prayers of my childhood brought me no comfort. I often called out to God because I thought at least He couldn't be taken away, but there was no response from His direction. It became apparent to me that I was truly a bad person and that was why my calls went unheard.

The only way I knew how to cope with my emptiness, isolation, and pain was to dissociate and leave my body. When the pain became too great, I was able to remove myself by either floating up around the ceiling, sitting on a shelf in a corner of the room, or crawling into the center of a flower that was on the wallpaper in the room.

Yet something has kept me alive, refusing to give up, to give in. My ambassador would quickly say that like Frankl, it is because my inner life has become more and more intense and that without always knowing it, I have been struggling for a long time to find meaning. So that, like Frankl, my spirit could pierce through this hopeless and meaningless existence in order to find a purpose for my life.

Until I began my work with Dr. S., I was more afraid of living than of dying. I had lost faith that there really was a future for me. I felt trapped in the hole of deep despair. Little by little, I am coming to experience a different sense about what is possible even for me. Nietzsche wrote, "He who has a why to live for can bear with almost any how." I feel that I am living proof of this statement and my ambassador is helping me understand that I am worthwhile, that I am salvageable.

Frankl speaks again and again about love. I have always been uncomfortable with the word love. But my ambassador wants me to know that what we [my ambassador and I] have experienced in this therapeutic process is a love and tenderness that we have not known before and that it is deeply mutual. There is a mutual care, trust, and respect that has enabled me to call up my therapist [activation of a positive therapist introject] in situations that have been difficult and painful, when I didn't know how to help myself. Just as Frankl was able to call up the image of his wife, I can now picture my companions' faces [those of my psychologist, psychiatrist, and spiritual leader] and hear them giving me words of encouragement and experience them staying with me so that I can come to experience a better outcome. They continue to help strengthen my mental courage as well as point out that while I cannot change the past, I can speak up for the present. It is because of them that I can walk down the street holding my head up instead of always looking down. That I can listen to music and allow myself to be moved by the sound of an oboe, a sound that speaks plainly to my heart, or truly see the color of a flower and the veins in its petals. Like Frankl, I have come to understand the importance of seeing beauty in the midst of the ugliness of life.

Frankl speaks of turning personal tragedy and suffering into inner achievement and that this suffering ceases at the moment it finds meaning. I cannot change what has happened, but I continue to work on changing myself. All that I have and continue to learn hopefully moves me closer to being a source of help and comfort to those who suffer.

My ambassador says that I am continuing to find my voice and that I have something worthwhile to say. What I have accomplished no one can take away, and what will follow can only strengthen who I am becoming. It is because I have experienced love and the ability to love in return that I am able to continue my commitment to this process. Just as Frankl was able to picture his beloved wife, I too can picture these significant people in my life and realize that I am no longer alone to tough out this journey. I am grateful and owe my life to them. I continue to say "yes" to the search for meaning and know that the best is yet to come.

APPENDICES

Appendix A: Treatment Rationale

A copy of this Appendix is given to the client at the end of the first session.

> When we undergo a trauma, we experience a sense of extreme danger, whether physical, emotional, or both. The natural response to such an event is intense fear, which involves urges to fight, flee, or freeze. These responses are normal, automatic reactions to danger. They can affect our bodies (e.g., heart pounding, sweating), our thoughts (e.g., thinking we are in danger), and our actions (e.g., trying to get away). These intense responses can reoccur years after the trauma if something in our lives triggers memories of the event.
>
> All aspects of your traumatic experience exist in a network of memories. Body sensations, odors, time of day or night, or the place in which the trauma occurred may all become part of this memory. It is like a "fear network" in your mind.
>
> If you think about the traumatic event or see something reminding you of it, you may experience intense feelings of fear, disgust, guilt, shame, rage, or sorrow—much like what you felt at the time of the trauma. Reexperiencing these feelings causes great distress, which is why most people try to push away these painful memories or ignore them. You may

tell yourself, "I should just forget about the whole thing and not let it bother me anymore," or "If I don't think about it, it will eventually go away."

Some people may try to convince you that avoidance is the best way to cope with trauma. Friends, relatives, or even partners may feel uncomfortable hearing about your experience and discourage you from talking about it. Unfortunately, trying to ignore your feelings and fears does not make them go away. Often the traumatic event comes back to haunt you through painful recurring memories, flashbacks, or nightmares because it is "unfinished business."

As you know from your own experience, it is not easy to recover from childhood traumas. How you view yourself, others, and the world in general has been dramatically affected by your trauma. You may find it difficult to believe in yourself or to trust anyone. We are here to help you with this.

The purpose of our work together here is to help you work through, and move beyond, your traumatic memories. We have found that this treatment not only helps people like yourself overcome trauma-related memories, it also helps them to develop a healthier self-image and to move forward with their lives as "thrivers."

Much of the work we will be doing involves the use of imagery or visualization. The therapy involves asking you to visually recall and reexperience the traumatic images, thoughts, and feelings you experience during a flashback (or nightmare). Initially, I will ask you to visualize the entire memory in imagery as you remember it. Then we will go back over it again and this time change, or rescript, the imagery to create a better outcome for you, one that leaves you feeling more empowered and in control. The aim is to replace your victimization images with mastery images so that you can see and feel yourself responding to your trauma no longer as a victim, but as an empowered individual. This, of course, does not change the traumatic events themselves, but it can change the lingering images, thoughts, feelings, and beliefs that you have about the trauma.

Appendix B: The Post-Imagery Questionnaire (PIQ)

The PIQ was developed by the senior author for use with survivors of childhood abuse who continue to be haunted by visual recurring memories of their traumas. The PIQ is administered to the patient following an imagery rescripting session as a means of obtaining immediate and direct client feedback about the session just experienced. The PIQ consists of two forms, PIQ-A and PIQ-B. While some overlap exists between the two forms, specific items vary in accordance with the particular phase of rescripting that the client is in at the moment.

The PIQ-A is administered immediately after imagery sessions conducted during imagery phase I, which involve both the imaginal exposure (reexperiencing the abuse imagery) and the mastery imagery components (sessions 1 to 8 in the standard protocol). The PIQ-B is administered immediately after imagery sessions conducted during imagery phase II, which involve ADULT–CHILD imagery only (after session 8 in the standard protocol).

The PIQ-A is designed to obtain a quick and ongoing cognitive assessment of the abuse victim's schematic shift from maladaptive abuse-related beliefs to more adaptive beliefs in the following areas:

1. from self-perceived powerlessness to self-empowerment vis-à-vis the perpetrator,
2. from self-directed anger to perpetrator-directed anger,
3. from self-directed blame to perpetrator-directed blame,
4. from self-hatred to self-acceptance,
5. from an inability to self-nurture to a significantly enhanced ability to self-nurture.

Once the abuse victim no longer feels helpless and powerless vis-à-vis the perpetrator—as reflected by the presence of empowering mastery imagery that can be visualized with relative ease—the focus of rescripting then shifts to confronting the victim's negative self-schemas through imaginal ADULT–CHILD interactions. The PIQ-B is thus designed to obtain an ongoing cognitive assessment of the abuse victim's schematic shift in the following areas:

1. from self-directed anger, self-hatred, and self-blame to self-acceptance;
2. from feeling disconnected and abandoned to feeling a sense of connectedness;
3. from feeling untrusting and unsafe with oneself to feeling more trusting and safe with oneself;
4. from perceived fragmentation of the ADULT and CHILD parts of self to a healthier accommodation and integration of the ADULT and CHILD.

ADMINISTRATION OF THE PIQ

The PIQ is designed to be administered by the clinician immediately following the completion of an imagery session. The clinician introduces the PIQ to the client as follows:

I would like to ask you a few questions about the imagery session we just completed. I will be asking you to rate your response to each item on a 0 to 100 scale. Do you need a few moments to get reoriented?

Once the client has indicated a readiness to begin, the clinician reads aloud the items of the PIQ-A beginning with item 1:

On a scale of 0 to 100, how vivid was the imagery you experienced during our session today? Zero would indicate that you could not develop the imagery at all, and 100 would indicate that the imagery was extremely vivid.

After recording the client's response on the line to the left of item 1, the clinician then proceeds to item 2 following the same procedure until all items have been administered.

SCORING AND INTERPRETATION OF THE PIQ

When the client's responses to all of the PIQ items have been recorded, the clinician notes the items with an asterisk (*) next to them. These are reversed items and their real scores are computed in the following manner:

Where x equals the reported client rating score
(i.e., the actual number reported on a reversed item),
$100 - x$ = real item score.

The real item score of each item without an asterisk is the actual number reported by the client. The total PIQ score is then calculated by obtaining the sum of all individual real item scores of items 1 to 10. (Items A and B of both PIQ forms are not tabulated in the total PIQ score.)

Total scores in each PIQ form range from 0 to 1,000. The higher the total PIQ score, the more acute is the degree of abuse-related cognitive dysfunctionality and affective distress. As the imagery sessions progress, a significant drop in the total PIQ scores should be noted. Although the PIQ appears to have good face validity, psychometric data are not yet available for either form.

POST-IMAGERY QUESTIONNAIRE–A (PIQ-A)

Name of Client: _____ Date: _____

After each mastery session, ask the client to rate on a 0 to 100 scale the following:

Client Rating   *Real Score*

_____ *A. How *vivid* was the imagery you   _____
           experienced during our session today?

    0 = Could not develop imagery at all
  100 = Extremely vivid

_____ B. How much did you mentally escape or   _____
           dissociate during the imagery?

    0 = Did not mentally escape or dissociate
        at all during the imagery
  100 = Mentally escaped or dissociated so
        much that you could not stay with
        the imagery.

- -

_____ 1. How *afraid* were you, the ADULT,   _____
          of confronting the perpetrator?

    0 = Not at all afraid of confronting
        the perpetrator
  100 = Extremely afraid (as afraid as   _____
        you have ever felt)

_____ *2. How much *anger* did you, the ADULT,   _____
           feel towards the perpetrator?

    0 = No anger at all
  100 = Extreme anger (as angry as you
        have ever felt toward anyone)

Client Rating   ***Real Score***

_____ 3. How *powerless* did you, the ADULT,   _____
          feel when confronting the
          perpetrator?

          0 =   Felt very empowered
          100 = Felt extremely helpless and
                powerless

_____ 4. How difficult was it for you,   _____
          the ADULT, to *rescue* the CHILD?

          0 =   Not at all difficult (able to
                rescue the CHILD without
                difficulty)
          100 = Extremely difficult
                (unable to rescue the CHILD
                without help)

_____ *5. How much did you, the ADULT, feel   _____
          the perpetrator was to *blame* for the
          abuse?

          0 =   Did not blame the perpetrator
                at all for the abuse
          100 = Felt the perpetrator was totally
                to blame for the abuse

_____ 6. How much did you, the ADULT, feel   _____
          the CHILD was to *blame* for the
          abuse?

          0 =   Did not feel the CHILD was at
                all to blame for the abuse
          100 = Felt the CHILD was totally to
                blame for the abuse

THE POST-IMAGERY QUESTIONNAIRE (PIQ)

Client Rating   ***Real Score***

_____ 7. How much *anger* did you, the ADULT, feel towards the CHILD? _____

       0 = No anger at all

       100 = Extreme anger (as angry as you have ever felt toward anyone)

_____ *8. How difficult was it for you, the ADULT, to *nurture* the CHILD? _____

       0 = Unable to nurture the CHILD at all

       100 = Able to nurture the CHILD without difficulty

_____ *9. How *accepting* was the CHILD of you, the ADULT? _____

       0 = Not at all accepting

       100 = Totally accepting

_____ *10. How *safe* did the CHILD feel with you, the ADULT? _____

       0 = Not at all safe

       100 = Totally safe

Total PIQ Score _____

POST-IMAGERY QUESTIONNAIRE–B (PIQ-B)

Name of Client: _____ Date: _____

After each mastery session, ask the client to rate on a 0 to 100 scale the following:

Client Rating   *Real Score*

_____ *A. How *vivid* was the imagery you   _____
        experienced during our session today?

        0 = Could not develop imagery at all
        100 = Extremely vivid

_____ B. How much did you mentally escape or   _____
        dissociate during the imagery?

        0 = Did not mentally escape or dissociate
            at all during the imagery
        100 = Mentally escaped or dissociated so
            much that you could not stay with
            the imagery.

_____ *1. How *close* (in distance) were you, the _____
        ADULT, to the CHILD at the
        beginning of the imagery?

        0 = Not at all close
        100 = Very close

_____ 2. How *abandoned* was the CHILD   _____
        feeling at the beginning of the
        imagery?

        0 = Felt not at all abandoned
        100 = Felt extremely abandoned

THE POST-IMAGERY QUESTIONNAIRE (PIQ)

Client Rating   ***Real Score***

____   3. How difficult was it for you, the
           ADULT, to physically *approach*
           the CHILD?   ____

      0 = Able to approach the CHILD
           without difficulty

    100 = Felt unable to approach the
           CHILD

____   *4. How *connected* did you, the
           ADULT, feel with the CHILD
           by the end of the imagery
           session?   ____

      0 = Felt unable to connect with the
           CHILD at all

    100 = Felt very connected with the
           CHILD

____   5. How *abandoned* was the CHILD
           feeling by the end of the imagery
           session?   ____

      0 = Felt not at all abandoned

    100 = Felt extremely abandoned

____   6. How much did you, the ADULT,
           feel the CHILD was to *blame*
           for the abuse?   ____

      0 = Did not feel the CHILD
           was at all to blame for
           the abuse

    100 = Felt the CHILD was totally to
           blame for the abuse

Client Rating   **Real Score**

____   7. How much *anger* did you, the ADULT, feel toward the CHILD?   ____

       0 = Felt no anger at all toward the CHILD

       100 = Felt extreme anger toward the CHILD

____   8. How difficult was it for you, the ADULT, to *nurture* the CHILD?   ____

       0 = Able to nurture the CHILD without difficulty

       100 = Unable to nurture the CHILD

____   *9. How *accepting* was the CHILD of you, the ADULT, by the end of the imagery session?   ____

       0 = Not at all accepting

       100 = Totally accepting

____   *10. How *safe* did the CHILD feel with you, the ADULT, by the end of the imagery session?   ____

       0 = Not at all safe

       100 = Totally safe

                                     Total PIQ Score   ____

Appendix C: Therapist Record

Name of Client: _____ Date: _____
Name of Therapist: _____ Imagery Session #: _____
Homework Compliance/Problems/Comments: _____
_____
Description of Imaginal Exposure: _____
_____
Description of Mastery Imagery: _____
_____
Description of ADULT–CHILD Imagery: _____
_____

SUDs Ratings (Subjective Units of Discomfort 0 to 100) During:

	Imaginal Exposure	Mastery Imagery	ADULT–CHILD Imagery
Beginning (SUDs)	_____	_____	_____
10 minutes (SUDs)	_____	_____	_____
20 minutes (SUDs)	_____	_____	_____
30 minutes (SUDs)	_____	_____	_____
40 minutes (SUDs)	_____	_____	_____
50 minutes (SUDs)	_____	_____	_____
60 minutes (SUDs)	_____	_____	_____

Comments:

Appendix D: Homework Record

Name of Therapist: _____   Date: _____

Name of Client: _____   Session #: _____

Homework Assignment: Listen daily to audiotape of entire imagery session (exposure and rescripting).

Record **Subjective Units of Distress (SUDs: 0 to 100)** at the beginning and end of listening to the audiotape.

Self-administer the **Post-Imagery Questionnaire** (PIQ-A or PIQ-B) immediately after listening to the tape and record the PIQ score.

Day	1	2	3	4	5	6	7
Date and Time							
SUDs Beginning							
SUDs Ending							
SUDs Peak							
PIQ Score (A or B)							

Day	8	9	10	11	12	13	14
Date and Time							
SUDs Beginning							
SUDs Ending							
SUDs Peak							
PIQ Score (A or B)							

Appendix E: Traumatic Flashback Incident Record

PRETREATMENT

Name of Client: **Date:**

Number	Recurring Flashback	Duration	Frequency Daily Weekly	Peak SUDs (0–100)
1				
2				
3				
4				
5				

Number	Recurring Nightmare	Duration	Frequency Daily Weekly	Peak SUDs (0–100)
1				
2				
3				
4				
5				

TRAUMATIC FLASHBACK INCIDENT RECORD

SESSION # ____

Name of Client: _____ **Date:** _____

Number	Recurring Flashback	Duration	Frequency Daily Weekly	Peak SUDs (0–100)
1				
2				
3				
4				
5				

Number	Recurring Nightmare	Duration	Frequency Daily Weekly	Peak SUDs (0–100)
1				
2				
3				
4				
5				

TRAUMATIC FLASHBACK INCIDENT RECORD

POSTTREATMENT

Name of Client: Date:

Number	Recurring Flashback	Duration	Frequency Daily Weekly	Peak SUDs (0–100)
1				
2				
3				
4				
5				

Number	Recurring Nightmare	Duration	Frequency Daily Weekly	Peak SUDs (0–100)
1				
2				
3				
4				
5				

TRAUMATIC FLASHBACK INCIDENT RECORD

FOLLOW-UP————MONTHS

Name of Client: Date:

Number	Recurring Flashback	Duration	Frequency Daily Weekly	Peak SUDs (0–100)
1				
2				
3				
4				
5				

Number	Recurring Nightmare	Duration	Frequency Daily Weekly	Peak SUDs (0–100)
1				
2				
3				
4				
5				

References

American Psychiatric Association (1994). *Diagnostic and Statistical Manual of Mental Disorders*, 4th ed. Washington, DC: Author.

Bagley, C., and Ramsay, R. (1986). Disrupted childhood and vulnerability to sexual assault: long-term sequels with implications for counselling. *Social Work and Human Sexuality* 4:33–48.

Beck, A. T. (1976). *Cognitive Therapy and the Emotional Disorders*. New York: International Universities Press.

Beck, A. T., Emery, G., and Greenberg, R. L. (1985). *Anxiety Disorders and Phobias: A Cognitive Perspective*. New York: Basic Books.

Beck, A. T., Freeman, A., and Associates (1990). *Cognitive Therapy of Personality Disorders*. New York: Basic Books.

Beck, A. T., Rush, A. J., Shaw, B. F., and Emery, G. (1979). *Cognitive Therapy of Depression*. New York: Guilford.

Beck, A. T., Ward, C. H., Mendelson, M., et al. (1961). An inventory for measuring depression. *Archives of General Psychiatry* 4:561–571.

Bernstein, E. M., and Putnam, F. W. (1986). Development, reliability, and validity of a dissociation scale. *Journal of Nervous and Mental Disorders* 174:727–734.

Bettelheim, B. (1984). Afterword. In *I Didn't Say Good-bye*, ed. C. Vegh, pp. 165–167. New York: Dutton.

Beutler, L., Williams, R., and Zetzer, H. (1994). Efficacy of treatment for victims of child sexual abuse. *The Future of Children: Sexual Abuse of Children* 4(2):156–175.

Binet, A. (1922). *L'etude experimentale de l'intelligence.* Paris: Costes.

Blake-White, J., and Kline, C. M. (1985). Treating the dissociative process in adult victims of childhood incest. *Social Casework: The Journal of Contemporary Social Work* 9:394–402.

Bowlby, J. (1988). *A Secure Base: Parent–Child Attachment and Healthy Human Development.* New York: Basic Books.

Bretherton, I. (1987). New perspectives on attachment relations in infancy: security, communication and internal working models. In *Handbook of Infant Development*, 2nd ed., ed. J. D. Osofsky, pp. 1061–1100. New York: Wiley.

Breuer, J., and Freud, S. (1895/1955). Studies on hysteria. *Standard Edition* 2:1–305.

Briere, J. (1989). *Therapy for Adults Molested as Children: Beyond Survival.* New York: Springer.

—— (1992). *Child Abuse Trauma: Theory and Treatment of the Lasting Effects.* Newbury Park, CA: Sage.

—— (1995). *Trauma symptom inventory professional manual.* Odessa, FL: Psychological Assessment Resources.

—— (1997a). *Psychological assessment of adult posttraumatic states.* Washington, DC: American Psychological Association.

—— (1997b). Psychological assessment of interpersonal victimization effects in adults and children. *Psychotherapy: Theory, Research and Practice* 34(4):353–364.

Briere, J., and Runtz, M. (1987). Post sexual abuse trauma: data and implications for clinical practice. *Journal of Interpersonal Violence* 2:367–379.

—— (1992). The long-term effects of sexual abuse: a review and synthesis. In *Treating Victims of Child Sexual Abuse*, ed. J. Briere, pp. 3–14. San Francisco: Jossey-Bass.

Browne, A., and Finkelhor, D. (1986). Impact of child sexual abuse: a review of the research. *Psychological Bulletin* 99:66–77.

Bruner, J. (1973). *Beyond the Information Given.* New York: Norton.

Bryer, J. B., Nelson, B. A., Miller, J. B., and Krol, P. A. (1987). Childhood sexual and physical abuse as factors in adult psychiatric illness. *American Journal of Psychiatry* 144:1426–1430.

Carlson, E. B. (1996). *Trauma Assessments: A Clinician's Guide.* New York: Guilford.

Carlson, E. B., and Putnam, F. W. (1993). An update on the Dissociative Experiences Scale. *Dissociation* 6:16–27.

Clark, D. M. (1986). A cognitive approach to panic. *Behavior, Research, and Therapy* 24:461–470.

Coons, P. M., Bowman, E. S., Pellow, T. A., and Schneider, P. (1989). Post-traumatic aspects of the treatment of victims of sexual abuse and incest. *Psychiatric Clinics of North America* 12(2):325–335.

Courtois, C. A. (1988). *Healing the Incest Wound: Adult Survivors in Therapy.* New York: Norton.

——— (1996). Psychometric review of Incest History Questionnaire. In *Measurement of Stress, Trauma, and Adaptation,* ed. B. H. Stamm, pp. 189–191. Lutherville, MD: Sidran.

Dancu, C. V., Hearst-Ikeda, D., Foa, E. B., and Smucker, M. R. (in preparation). Treatment of chronic posttraumatic stress disorder in adult survivors of incest: cognitive/behavioral interventions.

Donaldson, M. A., and Gardner, R. (1985). Diagnosis and treatment of traumatic stress among women after childhood incest. In *Trauma and Its Wake,* vol. 1, ed. C. R. Figley, pp. 356–377. New York: Brunner/Mazel.

Edwards, D. J. A. (1990). Cognitive therapy and the restructuring of early memories through guided imagery. *Journal of Cognitive Psychotherapy: An International Quarterly* 4:33–51.

Edwards, P., and Donaldson, M. (1989). Assessment of symptoms in adult survivors of incest. *Child Abuse and Neglect* 13:101–110.

Elliott, D. M., and Briere, J. (1992). Sexual abuse trauma among professional women: validating the Trauma Symptom Checklist-40 (TSC-40). *Child Abuse and Neglect* 16:391–398.

Finkelhor, D. (1990). Early and long-term effects of child sexual abuse: an update. *Professional Psychology* 21:325–330.

Finkelhor, D., and Browne, A. (1985). The traumatic impact of child sexual abuse: a conceptualization. *American Journal of Orthopsychiatry* 55:530–541.

Finkelhor, D., Hotaling, G., Lewis, I. A., and Smith, C. (1989). Sexual abuse and its relationship to later sexual satisfaction, marital status, religion, and attitudes. *Journal of Interpersonal Violence* 4:279-299.

Foa, E. B. (1995). *Posttraumatic Stress Diagnostic Scale (PDS) manual.* Minneapolis, MN: National Computer Systems.

Foa, E. B., and Kozak, M. J. (1986). Emotional processing of fear: exposure to corrective information. *Psychological Bulletin* 99:20-35.

Foa, E. B., Riggs, D. S., Dancu, C. V., and Rothbaum, B. D. (1993). Reliability and validity of a brief instrument assessing posttraumatic stress disorder. *Journal of Traumatic Stress* 6:459-474.

Foa, E. B., Rothbaum, B. O., Riggs, D. S., and Murdock, T. B. (1991). Treatment of post-traumatic stress disorder in rape victims: a comparison between cognitive-behavioral procedures and counseling. *Journal of Consulting and Clinical Psychology* 59:715-723.

Ford, J. D., Fisher, P., and Larson, L. (1997). Object relations as a predictor of treatment outcome with chronic posttraumatic stress disorder. *Journal of Consulting and Clinical Psychology* 65(4):547-559.

Frankl, V. E. (1959). *Man's Search for Meaning: An Introduction to Logotherapy.* New York: Simon & Schuster, 1984.

Friedrich, W. N. (1991). Sexual behavior in sexually abused children. In *Treating Victims of Child Sexual Abuse*, ed. J. N. Briere, pp. 15-28. San Francisco: Jossey-Bass.

Gomes-Schwartz, B., Horowitz, J. M., and Cardarelli, A. P. (1990). *Child Sexual Abuse: The Initial Effects.* Newbury Park, CA: Sage.

Goodwin, J., and Talwar, N. (1989). Group psychotherapy for victims of incest. *Psychiatric Clinics of North America: Treatment of Victims of Sexual Abuse* 12:257-278.

Grunert, B., Rusch, M., Smucker, M. R., and Mendelson, R. (in preparation). Imagery Rescripting treatment of PTSD in victims of industrial accidents following treatment failure with imaginal exposure.

Grunert, B., Weis, J., and Rusch, M. (in preparation). Early vs. delayed imaginal exposure for the treatment of PTSD following accidental injury.

Guidano, V. F. (1987). *Complexity of the Self.* New York: Guilford.

Guidano, V. F., and Liotti, G. (1983). *Cognitive Processes and Emotional Disorders: A Structural Approach to Psychotherapy*. New York: Guilford.

Harvey, J. J., Orbuch, T. L., Chwalisz, K. D., and Garwood, G. (1991). Coping with sexual assault: the role of account making and confiding. *Journal of Traumatic Stress* 4:515–532.

Henry, W. P., Schacht, T. E., and Strupp, H. H. (1990). Patient and therapist introject, interpersonal process, and differential psychotherapy outcome. *Journal of Consulting and Clinical Psychology* 58(6):768–774.

Herman, J. L. (1992). *Trauma and Recovery*. New York: Basic Books.

Horowitz, M. J. (1986). *Stress Response Syndromes*, 2nd ed. Northvale, NJ: Jason Aronson.

Janet, P. (1898). *Nervoses et idees fixes*. Paris: Alcan.

—— (1919). *Les medications psychologiques: Etudes historiques, psychologiques et cliniques sur les methodes de la psychotherapie*, vols. 1–3. Paris: Alcan.

Janoff-Bulman, R. (1985). The aftermath of victimization: rebuilding shattered assumptions. In *Trauma and Its Wake*, vol. 1, ed. C. R. Figley, pp. 15–35. New York: Brunner/Mazel.

—— (1989). Assumptive worlds and the stress of traumatic events: applications of the schema construct. *Social Cognition* 7:113–136.

—— (1996). Psychometric review of World Assumptions Scale. In *Measurement of Stress, Trauma, and Adaptation*, ed. B. H. Stamm, pp. 440–442. Lutherville, MD: Sidran.

Jehu, D. (1988). *Beyond Sexual Abuse: Therapy with Women Who Were Childhood Victims*. Chichester, UK: Wiley.

—— (1991). Posttraumatic stress reactions among adults molested as children. *Sexual and Marital Therapy* 6:227–243.

Jung, C. G. (1960). *The Structure and Dynamics of the Psyche*, trans. R. F. C. Hull. Princeton, NJ: Princeton University Press, 1926.

—— (1976). *The Symbolic Life*, trans. R. F. C. Hull. Princeton, NJ: Princeton University Press, 1935.

Kimerling, R., and Calhoun, K. S. (1994). Somatic symptoms, social support, and treatment seeking among sexual assault victims. *Journal of Consulting and Clinical Psychology* 62(2):333–340.

Kolko, D. J., Moser, J. T., and Weldy, S. R. (1988). Behavioral/emotional indications of sexual abuse in child psychiatric inpatients: a controlled comparison with physical abuse. *Child Abuse and Neglect* 12:529–542.

Kosbab, F. P. (1974). Imagery techniques in psychiatry. *Archives of General Psychiatry* 31:283–290.

Lang, P. J. (1979). A bio-informational theory of emotional imagery. *Psychophysiology* 16:495–512.

——— (1986). The cognitive psychophysiology of emotion: fear and anxiety. In *Anxiety and the Anxiety Disorders*, ed. A. H. Tuma and J. D. Maser, pp. 130–179. Hillsdale, NJ: Lawrence Erlbaum.

Leahy, R. L. (1996). *Cognitive Therapy: Basic Principles and Applications*. Northvale, NJ: Jason Aronson.

Lipovsky, J. A., Saunders, B. E., and Murphy, S. M. (1989). Depression, anxiety, and behavior problems among victims of father–child sexual assault and nonabused siblings. *Journal of Interpersonal Violence* 4:452–468.

Marmar, C. R., Weiss, D. S., and Metzler, T. J. (1996). The Peritraumatic Dissociative Experiences Questionnaire. In *Assessing Psychological Trauma and PTSD*, ed. J. Wilson and T. Keane, pp. 412–428. New York: Guilford.

McCann, I. L., and Pearlman, L. A. (1990). *Psychological Trauma and the Adult Survivor: Theory, Therapy, and Transformation*. New York: Brunner/Mazel.

McCann, I. L., Sakheim, D. K., and Abrahamson, D. J. (1988). Trauma and victimization: a model of psychological adaptation. *The Counseling Psychologist* 16:531–594.

Meichenbaum, D. (1993). Stress inoculation training: a twenty-year update. In *Principles and Practices of Stress Management*, ed. R. L. Woolfolk and P. M. Lehrer. New York: Guilford.

——— (1994). *A Clinical Handbook/Practical Therapist Manual: For Assessing and Treating Adults with Post-Traumatic Stress Disorder (PTSD)*. Waterloo, Ontario: Institute Press.

Moore, B. E., and Fine, B. D. (1990). *Psychoanalytic Terms and Concepts*. New Haven: Yale University Press.

Morrow, S. L., and Smith, M. L. (1995). Constructions of survival and coping by women who have survived childhood sexual abuse. *Journal of Counseling Psychology* 42(1):24–33.

National Victim Center and Crime Victims Research and Treatment Center (1992). *Rape in America: a report to the nation.* Research report #1992-1. Washington, DC.

Norris, F. H., and Perilla, J. (1996). Reliability, validity, and cross-language stability of the Revised Civilian Mississippi Scale for PTSD. *Journal of Traumatic Stress* 9:285–298.

North, C. S., Smith, E. M., and Spitznagel, E. L. (1994). Violence and the homeless: an epidemiologic study of victimization and aggression. *Journal of Traumatic Stress* 7:95–110.

O'Neill, K., and Gupta, K. (1991). Post-traumatic stress disorder in women who were victims of childhood sexual abuse. *Irish Journal of Psychological Medicine* 8(2):124–127.

Pearlman, L. A. (1996). Review of TSI Belief Scale, Revision-L. In *Measurement of Stress, Trauma, and Adaptation*, ed. B. H. Stamm. Lutherville, MD: Sidran.

Pennebaker, J. W. (1993). Putting stress into words: health, linguistic, and therapeutic implications. *Behavior Research and Therapy* 6:539–548.

Peterson, K. C., Prout, M. F., and Schwartz, R. A. (1991). *Post-Traumatic Stress Disorder: A Clinician's Guide.* New York: Plenum.

Rachman, S. (1980). Emotional processing. *Behavior Research and Therapy* 18:51–60.

Resick, P., and Schnicke, M. K. (1993). *Cognitive Processing Therapy for Rape Victims: A Treatment Manual.* Newbury Park, CA: Sage.

Rosen, H. (1989). Piagetian theory and cognitive therapy. In *Comprehensive Handbook of Cognitive Therapy*, ed. A. Freeman, K. M. Simon, L. E. Beutler, and H. Arkowitz, pp. 189–212. New York: Plenum.

Rothbaum, B. O., and Foa, E. B. (1992). Exposure therapy for rape victims with posttraumatic stress disorder. *The Behavior Therapist* 9:219–222.

Russell, D. E. H. (1986). *The Secret Trauma: Incest in the Lives of Girls and Women.* New York: Basic Books.

Silver, R. L., Boon, C., and Stones, M. H. (1983). Searching for meaning in misfortune: making sense of incest. *Journal of Social Issues* 39:81–102.

Smucker, M. R. (1997). Posttraumatic stress disorder. In *Practicing Cognitive Therapy*, ed. R. L. Leahy, pp. 193–220. Northvale, NJ: Jason Aronson.

Smucker, M. R., Dancu, C., and Foa, E. B. (1991). *A manual for the treatment of adult survivors of childhood sexual abuse suffering from posttraumatic stress.* Unpublished manuscript.

Smucker, M. R., Dancu, C., Foa, E. B., and Niederee, J. L. (1995). Imagery Rescripting: a new treatment for survivors of childhood sexual abuse suffering from posttraumatic stress. *Journal of Cognitive Psychotherapy: An International Quarterly* 9(1):3–17.

Smucker, M. R., and Niederee, J. (1995). Treating incest-related PTSD and pathogenic schemas through imaginal exposure and rescripting. *Cognitive and Behavioral Practice* 2:63–93.

Spielberger, C. D. (1982). *Manual for the State-Trait Anxiety Inventory.* Palo Alto, CA: Consulting Psychologists Press.

Spielberger, C. D., Gorsuch, R. L., and Lushene, R. E. (1970). *Manual for the State-Trait Anxiety Inventory (Self-Evaluation Questionnaire).* Palo Alto, CA: Consulting Psychologists Press.

Spitzer, R. L., Williams, J. B. W., Gibbon, M., and First, M. B. (1989). *Structured Clinical Interview for DSM-III-R.* New York: Biometrics Research Department, New York State Psychiatric Institute.

Stamm, B. H. (1996). *Measurement of Stress, Trauma, and Adaptation.* Lutherville, MD: Sidran.

Staton, J. (1990). Using nonverbal methods in the treatment of sexual abuse. In *Violence Hits Home: Comprehensive Treatment Approaches to Domestic Violence,* ed. S. M. Stith, M. B. Williams, and K. Rosen, pp. 210–228. New York: Springer.

Terr, L. C. (1991). Childhood traumas: an outline and overview. *American Journal of Psychiatry* 148:10–20.

van der Kolk, B. A. (1987). The psychological consequences of overwhelming life experience. In *Psychological Trauma,* ed. B. A. van der Kolk, pp. 1–30. Washington, DC: American Psychiatric Press.

van der Kolk, B. A., and van der Hart, O. (1989). Pierre Janet and the breakdown of adaptation in psychological trauma. *American Journal of Psychiatry* 146:1530–1540.

——— (1991). The intrusive past: the flexibility of memory and the engraving of trauma. *American Imago* 48:425–454.

Vardi, D. J., Fisler, R. E., and Koenen, K. (1994). *Qualitative aspects of traumatic and nontraumatic memories: a preliminary study*. Poster session presented at the 10th annual meeting of the International Society for Traumatic Stress Studies, Chicago, November.

Vreven, D. L., Gudanowski, D. M., King, L. A., and King, D. W. (1995). The Civilian Version of the Mississippi PTSD Scale: a psychometric evaluation. *Journal of Traumatic Stress* 8:91–109.

Walker, L. (1994). *Abused Women and Survivor Therapy*. Washington, DC: American Psychological Association.

Weiss, D. S., and Marmar, C. R. (1996). The Impact of Event Scale–Revised. In *Assessing Psychological Trauma and PTSD*, ed. J. P. Wilson and T. Keane, pp. 399–411. New York: Guilford.

Wolpe, J. (1958). *Psychotherapy by Reciprocal Inhibition*. Stanford, CA: Stanford University Press.

Young, J. (1994). *Cognitive Therapy for Personality Disorders: A Schema-Focused Approach*. Sarasota, FL: Professional Resource Press.

Index

Active imagination, 24
Adult-nurturing-child imagery
 session 1, 50–52
 session 2, 58–60
 session 8, 76–78
 session 9, 84–86
 session 10 to 12, 89–90
 session 18, 114–116
American Psychiatric
 Association, 10
Attachment theory, imagery
 and, 25–26
Audiotaped sessions, imagery
 rescripting difficulties,
 137–140

Bagley, C., 6
Beck, A. T., 8, 21, 24, 25, 36
Bernstein, E. M., 36
Bettelheim, B., 16
Beutler, L., 5
Binet, A., 24
Blake-White, J., 9
Bowlby, J., 25

Bretherton, I., 26
Breuer, J., 23
Briere, J., 5, 6, 9, 36, 146, 148
Browne, A., 6, 8
Bruner, J., 12
Bryer, J. B., 5

Calhoun, K. S., 6
Carlson, E. B., 36
Case studies
 extended sessions, 184–218
 1 session, 155–158
 8 session, 161–179
Childhood sexual abuse. *See
 also* Posttraumatic stress
 disorder (PTSD); Trauma
 consequences of, 5–6
 prevalence of, 5
 trauma-related beliefs and
  schemata, 6–8
Clark, D. M., 38
Cognitive-behavioral theory,
 imagery in, 24–25

Cognitive processing, secondary versus primary, imagery and, 27–28
Contraindications, 143–149
  arousal increases, 143–145
  dissociation, 147–149
  generalized emotional numbing, 145–147
  partial intrusive ideation, 149
Coons, P. M., 6, 9
Courtois, C. A., 6, 36
Crisis management
  posttreatment, session 18, 118–120
  session 8, 78

Dancu, C. V., xvi
Diagnostic and Statistical Manual of Mental Disorders (DSM-IV), PTSD characteristics and symptoms, 10–11
Dissociation, contraindications, 147–149
Donaldson, M. A., 9, 36

Edwards, D. J. A., 24
Edwards, P., 36
Elliott, D. M., 36
Emotional numbing, generalized, contraindications, 145–147
Emotional processing, PTSD, 13–15
Exposure, imaginal, session 1, 46–48

Fine, B. D., 23, 27
Finkelhor, D., 5, 6, 8, 187

Flashback incident record, 237–240
Flashback writing, session 3, 64–65
Foa, E. B., 13, 14, 15, 21, 36, 145
Ford, J. D., 26
Frankl, V., 107, 108, 216, 217
Freud, S., 22, 23, 27
Friedrich, W. N., 6

Gardner, R., 9
Generalized emotional numbing, contraindications, 145–147
Gomes-Schwartz, B., 6
Goodwin, J., 6
Grunert, B., xvii
Guidano, V. F., 8
Gupta, K., 5, 9

Harvey, J. J., 16
Henry, W. P., 26, 27, 79
Herman, J. L., 6
Homework record, 235
Horowitz, M. J., 14

Imagery rescripting and reprocessing therapy (IRRT), 21–29. *See also* Case studies; Session
  attachment theory and, 25–26
  cognitive-behavioral context, 24–25
  cognitive processing, secondary versus primary, 27–28
  contraindications, 143–149. *See also* Contraindications
  development of, 21–22
  goals of, 29

historical context, 22–24
object relations theory and
 introjects, 26–27
posttreatment assessment, 120
pretreatment evaluation,
 35–38
relapse
 prevention/maintenance
 sessions, 120–121
session 1, 41–56
session 2, 56–62
session 3, 62–65
session 4, 66–68
session 5, 69–70
session 6, 71–72
session 7, 72–74
session 8, 74–79
session 9, 83–88
sessions 10 to 12, 88–91
session 13, 91–94
session 14, 97–100
session 15, 101–107
session 16, 107–110
session 17, 111–113
session 18, 113–121
Imagery rescripting difficulties,
 135–140
 audiotaped sessions, 137–140
 IRRT suspension indications,
 135–136
 options in, 136–137
Imagery rescripting format,
 127–131
 session 1, 127
 session 2, 127–128
 session 3, 128–129
 session 4, 129
 session 5, 129–130

Imaginal exposure
 session 1, 46–48
 session 2, 58–60
Information-processing models,
 PTSD, 13
Introjects
 development of positive,
 session 8, 78–79
 imagery and, 26–27
Intrusive ideation, partial,
 contraindications, 149

Janet, P., 22
Janoff-Bulman, R., 6, 8, 36
Jehu, D., 6, 8, 9
Jung, C., 23, 24

Kimerling, R., 6
Kline, C. M., 9
Kolko, D. J., 6
Kosbab, F. P., 23
Kozak, M. J., 13, 14, 21

Lang, P. J., 14
Language transformation,
 trauma, 15–17
Letter to perpetrator
 session 2, 60–62
 session 4, 67–68
Liotti, G., 8
Lipovsky, J. A., 6

Marmar, C. R., 36
Mastery imagery
 session 1, 48–50
 session 2, 58–60
 session 8, 76
McCann, I. L., 6, 8
Medication, IRRT and, 37
Meichenbaum, D., 16, 17, 145

Memory, traumatic, nature of, 11–12
Moore, B. E., 23, 27
Morrow, S. L., 187

National Victim Center, 5
Niederee, J., 8, 25
Norris, F. H., 36
North, C. S., 9

Object relations theory, imagery and, 26–27
O'Neill, K., 5, 9

Partial intrusive ideation, contraindications, 149
Pearlman, L. A., 8, 36
Pennebaker, J. W., 17
Perilla, J., 36
Peterson, K. C., 25
Piaget, J., 6, 12, 14
Post-imagery processing, debriefing and, session 2, 60
Post-Imagery Questionnaire-A, 223–226, 227–229
Post-Imagery Questionnaire-B
  administration of, 53, 224–225
  design of, 223–224
  scoring and interpretation of, 225–226
  session 9, 86–87
  text of, 230–232
Posttraumatic stress disorder (PTSD)
  characteristics and symptoms, 10–11
  emotional processing, 13–15
  information-processing models of, 13
  pilot study outcome summary, xvi–xvii
  traumagenic schemas linked to, 8–10
Posttreatment assessment, imagery rescripting and reprocessing therapy (IRRT), 120
Posttreatment safety contract, session 18, 118
Pretreatment evaluation, IRRT, 35–38
Primary cognitive processing, secondary versus, imagery and, 27–28
Putnam, F. W., 36

Rachman, S., 13
Ramsay, R., 6
Rationale presentation
  session 1, 42–45
  text of statement, 221–222
Relapse prevention/maintenance sessions
  format for, 130–131
  IRRT, 120–121
Rescripting
  session 1, 48–50
  session 2, 58–60
Resick, P., 28
Rosen, H., 6
Rothbaum, B. O., 15
Runtz, M., 6, 9
Rusch, M., xvii
Russell, D. E. H., 6

Safety contracting
  IRRT, session 1, 54–55
  posttreatment safety contract, 118

INDEX

Schnicke, M. K., 28
Secondary cognitive processing, primary versus, imagery and, 27–28
Self-calming and self-soothing abilities, assessment of, session 1, 54
Session 1
  adult-nurturing-child imagery, development of, 50–52
  context of, 41–42
  homework, 55–56
  imaginal exposure, 46–48
  mastery imagery, rescripting, 48–50
  post-imagery questionnaire, 53
  processing and debriefing, 53–54
  rationale presentation, 42–45
  rationale text, 221–222
  safety contracting, 54–55
  self-calming and self-soothing abilities, 54
  subject units of distress, 45–46
Session 2, 56–62
  context of, 56–58
  homework, 61–62
  imaginal exposure, mastery imagery, and ADULT–CHILD imagery, 58–60
  letter to perpetrator, 60–62
  post-imagery processing and debriefing, 60
Session 3, 62–65
  context of, 62–64
  flashback writing, 64–65
  homework, 65
Session 4, 66–68
  context of, 66–67
  follow-up letter, 67–68
Session 5, 68–70
Session 6, 71–72
Session 7, 72–74
Session 8, 74–79
  ADULT–CHILD only imagery phase, criteria for progression to, 76–77
  context of, 75
  crisis management, 77
  exposure, mastery, and adult-child imagery follow-up, 76
  homework, 78–79
  introjects, development of positive, 78–79
Session 9, 83–88
  adult-nurturing-child imagery, 84–86
  context of, 83–84
  homework, 87–88
  Post-Imagery Questionnaire-B administration, 86–87
  processing and debriefing, 87–88
Sessions 10 to 12, 88–91
  adult-nurturing-child imagery, 89–90
  context of, 88–89
  homework, 90–91
  Post-Imagery Questionnaire-B administration, 90
  processing and debriefing, 90
Session 13, 91–94

adult-nurturing-child imagery, 92–94
  context of, 91–92
  homework, 93–94
Session 14, 97–100
  context of, 97–98
  homework, 99–100
  new treatment phase introduced, 98–100
Session 15, 101–107
  context of, 101–103
  homework, 107
  suffering, meaning of, 106–107
  traumagenic schema modification, 103–106
Session 16, 107–110
  context of, 107–108
  homework, 109–110
  suffering, meaning of patient's, 108–110
Session 17, 111–113
Session 18, 113–121
  additional sessions consideration, 117–118
  ADULT–CHILD imagery follow-up, 114–116
  context of, 113–114
  crisis management, posttreatment, 118–120
  homework, 119–120
  posttreatment safety contract, 118
  termination consideration, 116–117
Shakespeare, W., 16
Silver, R. L., 16
Smith, M. L., 187

Smucker, M. R., 6, 8, 10, 13, 15, 22, 25, 143, 144
Spielberger, C. D., 36
Spitzer, R. L., 36
Stamm, B. H., 36
Staton, J., 25
Subject units of distress, introduction of, 45–46

Talwar, N., 6
Termination, session 18, 116–117
Terr, L. C., 12
Therapist record, 233
Trauma
  beliefs and schemata related to, 6–8
  language transformation, 15–17
  PTSD and, 8–10
  type I versus type II, 12–13
Traumagenic schema modification, session 15, 103–106
Traumatic memory, nature of, 11–12

van der Hart, O., 11, 16, 24
van der Kolk, B. A., 9, 11, 16, 24
Vardi, D. J., 11
Vreven, D. L., 36

Walker, L., 6
Weis, J., xvii
Weiss, D. S., 36
Wolpe, J., 26

Young, J., 8